That Went Well

That Went Well

Adventures in
Caring for My Sister

TERRELL
HARRIS DOUGAN

HYPERION   NEW YORK

Copyright © 2009 Terrell Dougan

All rights reserved. No part of this book may be used or reproduced in any
manner whatsoever without the written permission of the Publisher.
Printed in the United States of America. For information address
Hyperion, 77 West 66th Street, New York, New York 10023-6298.

Library of Congress Cataloging-in-Publication Data is available upon request.

ISBN: 978-1-4013-2329-5

Hyperion books are available for special promotions, premiums,
or corporate training.
For details contact Michael Rentas,
Proprietary Markets, Hyperion, 77 West 66th Street, 12th floor,
New York, New York 10023, or call 212-456-0133.

Design by Victoria Hartman

FIRST EDITION

10   9   8   7   6   5   4   3   2   1

To all caring siblings of people
with disabilities everywhere.

Oh, Honey.
I know, I've been there, I am there now.
I will always be here and it's not going away.
I wake up every day, as you do, asking,
"What fresh hell is *this*?"
Call me up and come over
and we'll have a nice cup of tea together.
Well of *course* I'll lace it with something stronger.
We darn well deserve it.

Contents

Prologue		ix
1.	Lightning Strikes Twice	1
2.	I Try to Confess	13
3.	We Find Out the Truth	29
4.	Childhood's End	35
5.	College and Onward	49
6.	Tilting at Windmills	61
7.	The Spies Who Loved Community	74
8.	Eviction Is Such an Ugly Word	83
9.	Shall We Begin—Again?	104
10.	Travels with Mom	110
11.	Losses and Tantrums (Mine)	117
12.	Trying to Get a Life	129

13. Family Struggling Please Help   140

14. Adventures in Community Life   157

15. Confessions of a Codependent   165

16. Bowling with Irene   173

17. Travels with Irene   182

18. Friends, Labels, and the Future   192

19. Letter to Irene   202

20. With a Big Surprise Ending   205

    Acknowledgments   209

Prologue

It's Christmastime, and in a bright supermarket, with "Joy to the World" spilling out of the overhead speaker, I am ducking a flying packaged chicken that is sailing past my head, thrown at me by my furious sister. I know the reason, of course. She doesn't want the vegetables I have put in the cart; she wants chocolate bars and a case of Coke for dinner.

As the chicken flies by, it stops the meat department cold. People are staring at us both, two middle-aged women, one throwing and one ducking the chicken. I want to say to them, Listen: she is mentally disabled, see? She can't read or write. She's diabetic, and can't have candy and Coke. We're doing the best we can here. If you'll just put down your meat for a minute, I'll tell you all about it. . . .

That Went Well

1

Lightning Strikes Twice

March 1946

It's late afternoon. The clouds are rolling in, swift and dark, and my grandmother, Bammy, and I hear the rumble of thunder. The willow tree branches sway as the wind kicks up. "Oh my, look at that," Bammy says, wrapping her arms around me as lightning flashes across the sky. It's a blustery, scary, stormy day: just the way we like it, especially since we're cuddled up safe and warm in the lamplight, with a coal fire burning in the fireplace. I am thinking of the pickled pigs' feet we'll eat while listening to our favorite radio program, *Mr. Keene, Tracer of Lost Persons.* Now the thunder claps so loudly it makes us jump. We both love the light show.

With one more deafening crack, thunder and lightning hit simultaneously, and our willow tree is smoking. Bammy screams and grabs me off the couch and into the middle of the living room. She's afraid the tree will fall through the window on us.

But it doesn't. It has split right down the middle, and the other half has fallen away from the house, toward the street.

Bammy runs to the telephone in the hall to call my dad. "Oh, Dick! The worst thing—yes, we're all right, but the willow tree just got struck by lightning and split right in two! And our lights all went off! Yes! Oh good, we'll see you in a few minutes."

When my father got home, the storm had died down. He stood there regarding the tree for a long time, his arms folded over his chest. Coming inside, he took off his coat and tie, put on blue jeans and a work shirt, and drove our 1945 Packard to the hardware store. He came back with a jar of black, tarlike goop to paint onto the trunk of the tree. "We're going to see if this will heal its wound and let it live and grow. It's still a pretty tree, even like this."

My little sister Irene had been born that morning, and Mom was still in the hospital. Since our electricity was out, we couldn't hear *Mr. Keene, Tracer of Lost Persons*, and we were sad about that. We ate our pickled pigs' feet by candlelight, which was okay, because we liked them cold just as well.

I had no idea then how much Irene's birth would change all our lives, irrevocably and forever.

The next day I sat on the couch and watched the tree people chop up the stricken half of the willow and haul it away. Bammy was on the phone with one of her friends: "Yes, the baby's here! Oh, Afton was in labor for hours. The doctor was mean to her, and her with her arthritis. . . . She had a terrible time. He made her put her feet in those stirrups when she couldn't bend her knees! Told her she was being a bad patient. I could kill that man! Oh yes, the baby's beautiful. They named her after me, you know. Yes! Irene! Well, tickled pink, of course."

When Mom came home with my new baby sister, I couldn't wait to hold Irene. She was beautiful and dainty, and fit in my arms like she belonged there. I loved her instantly, and of course so did Bammy, who crooned lullabies to her the way she had to me.

Mom and Dad slept in twin beds in a bedroom wallpapered in small pink roses and blue ribbons. Cuddling with Mom in that bed was my favorite thing to do. I loved her hands holding my arms. I thought her hands were beautiful: always perfectly manicured, the fingers splaying out sideways from hugely swollen knuckles. I wondered why mine didn't do that, and why Dad's and Bam's weren't as pretty as Mom's.

Mom would come home from a dinner party and sit on my bed if I was still awake. I loved the smell of her perfumes: Fleur de Rocaille or Joy. She would stroke my hair and tell me about the party. I always loved hearing about it until she came to the part where someone squeezed her swollen, arthritic hand. "Oh, it hurt so much! They don't know how my hands hurt, and they take them and squeeze them. It almost makes me *cry*, it hurts so much."

Then she would kiss me and go to her bedroom, leaving me furious at the person who squeezed my mother's hand and hurt her. She was so delicate. It made me want to protect her, and I was too little to do that.

But now she was home with Irene, who slept in a bassinet by Mom's bed so she could nurse her in the night. I wished I could crawl in with Mom and Irene so I would be safe, and so I could see the roses and ribbons on the wallpaper in the morning.

One night I waited until everyone had gone to bed, then crept into Bammy's bedroom next door to mine. She had just tuned in to her other favorite radio show, *True Detective,* "where real crimes are solved by real detectives, with real criminals brought to justice." She was rubbing cream on her heels.

"Bammy, have you noticed about Irene, that her eyes are crossed?"

"Yes, honey, I noticed."

"What's wrong, do you think?"

She put her jar of cream down and rubbed the rest into her hands. She frowned a little, thinking what to say, and then brightened. "Some babies get born that way and it takes a few months for the eyes to straighten out, that's all. Their muscles are just weak."

Bammy was my go-to person whenever I had questions. Mom didn't give answers as fun and colorful as Bammy's. While Mom had been pregnant, I asked how long it takes for a baby to get born. It was clear to me that you got married first and then you ordered one like you ordered up your newspaper delivery. Bammy thought a few moments and then said, "The first baby can come anytime after you're married. After that, it takes nine months."

Here are more facts she taught me:

1. If you stay in the bathtub too long and your fingers wrinkle up, it means you are going to dissolve and you have to get out immediately.
2. If you put your nightgown on inside out, you have to go to bed in it that way. If you change it, it's very bad luck, and when you die, you'll have to pick every stitch out of that nightgown with your teeth while you're in heaven. Bammy's mother, who was born in England in 1849, told her that. Everyone in her mom's village knew that rule for a fact.

3. Dreams go by opposites. If you dream about a death, it means a new baby is coming. And vice versa.

Bammy was my other mother, really, and my friend and my protector. She wasn't about to alarm us both with Irene's crossed eyes.

In the coming months, Irene's eyes weren't the only thing that seemed strange to me. Most days, Irene would lie quietly in her playpen, rotating her wrist round and round, watching her hand with fascination. I had never seen a baby do this before. Mrs. Murphy, across the field behind us, had just had her third baby, and none of them had ever acted that way. Besides, the other kids had learned to sit up by themselves faster than Irene did. Once she finally did sit up, Irene kept doing that thing with her hand. I could never figure it out. I mean, it seemed to me, once you've seen your hand, you've seen it. But to Irene, it was endlessly fascinating.

She was slow to do everything. When she finally walked at a year and a half, Tommy Murphy, who was playing with us in our sandpile, said, "Hey, what's wrong with your sister? How come it took her so long to walk?"

I looked at Tommy for a minute, trying to decide how to reply. "Nothing. She's just a little slow, that's all." I had heard my parents and Bammy say that over and over, looking at each other, hoping.

I hated the idea that Tommy noticed that there was something wrong with Irene, because the Murphys were everything I wanted our family to be: big, informal, and gloriously chaotic. I would go through the backyard from our Cape Cod home, past our vegetable garden, past the chicken coop and the sandpile and the swings, through the picket fence and the field, and into the Murphys' back lawn, where Mary Frances, Tommy, Grace Ann, and Margaret were playing. Mrs. Murphy was never in the yard. She always seemed to be pregnant and in the kitchen of their tiny, packed house, cooking and mumbling "Hail, Mary, full of grace," to herself, a cigarette hanging from her lips. That, for me, was where all the action was.

The Murphys were Catholics. Their house, clanking and buzzing with the messy clamor of laughing children, attracted me as a moth to a lightbulb. Toys lay on top of folded laundry in baskets. Someone was always chasing someone else: the game went on all day. Our swing set, sandpile, and chicken coop brought them all over to our backyard, too. My dad had planted a Victory Garden, which many Americans did during World War II, to be more self-sufficient. Dad also raised chickens. The Murphy kids used to love watching Bammy on a Sunday, going out to the chicken coop with her hatchet, grabbing the fattest hen she could find, and chopping its head off. We stood in wonder as it ran around for a few more minutes before its legs got the message.

The Murphy kids went to a private Catholic school. My friend Mary Frances told me she was going to be a nun when she grew up. I didn't believe it for a minute. I couldn't picture her in that penguin uniform they wore.

I always wanted to stay for dinner at the Murphys' house because it was so different from mine. First, Mrs. Murphy had us hold out our spoons. She went around the table filling each one with cod-liver oil, which I found very tasty. Then we folded our hands and said, "Bless us, O Lord, and these thy gifts. . . ." Dinner was often spaghetti with the best sauce I'd ever tasted, and then, glory of glories, Jell-O for dessert. Mom and Bammy never made Jell-O.

At my house when we had spaghetti, it was very different. I would push mine around on the plate, and when asked why I wasn't eating it, I would say, "I like Mrs. Murphy's better."

Mom considered herself the spaghetti queen; her gourmet sauce took an hour to prepare and a few more hours to simmer. When Irene and I were babies, she made us spaghetti with bacon, canned tomatoes, and Velveeta cheese. But for the family and guests, her big, meaty, grown-up spaghetti, laden with garlic, just a touch of sugar, and the secret ingredient, grated lemon peel, was the recipe all her friends copied. So naturally she was quite hurt that I preferred Mrs. Murphy's spaghetti sauce, and wondered if it was a big family secret.

Mom called Catherine Murphy to ask for her spaghetti sauce recipe. Catherine took a big puff on her cigarette and said, "I'm not going to tell you."

She had tasted Mom's spaghetti. She wasn't about to tell Mom she just poured a can of undiluted tomato soup over noodles.

To Mrs. Murphy, my family probably lived like royalty. Mom and Bam served elegant meals at our dinner table, laid with fresh flowers, crystal, and silver. My parents and my grandmother dressed up and went out a lot: Bammy to her bridge games, Mom and Dad to dinner parties. I have a memory of Mrs. Murphy, a wistful look on her face, balancing a baby on one hip, visiting our backyard as Mom laid embroidered white tablecloths and candles over card tables for a party that evening. Mrs. Murphy didn't realize it, but for me, her house was a running party, all day, every day. She didn't need any special settings: her big family *was* the party.

One summer evening Mrs. Murphy was standing at the top

of the steps on their back porch, watering the lawn with a hose. A baby was perched on her hip. Mr. Murphy, coming home from work, trudged up the hill from the bus stop, wearing his brown suit, and carrying his briefcase. As he approached, Mrs. Murphy very calmly and slowly turned the hose on him, drenching him completely, including his brown felt hat. There was no expression on her face. Mr. Murphy stood there dripping, looking back at her with no expression on his face, either. Mrs. Murphy, looking grave, turned the hose back to the lawn as if nothing had happened. We all stood stock still, staring.

Finally Mr. Murphy put down his soaked briefcase and started to shake with laughter. He ran up the stairs after Mrs. Murphy, who had dropped the hose and run with the baby into the house. Tommy grabbed the hose and showered us all as we scattered, squealing, across the yard. All I could think of was that my family would never have had that much fun in a month of summer evenings. Looking back on it, I can see that any woman might want to turn a hose on a man for whom she had borne six children in eight years.

Summer evenings at our house, my father's parents or Mom's brother Bob and his wife, Nicky, would drop in for a cocktail on the back patio. Uncle Bob, tall and handsome, and Aunt Nicky, who looked just like Vivien Leigh, completed our Sunday dinners. It was so pleasant: clinking ice cubes; the scent of freshly mown grass and roses in bloom against the white garage wall; Irene playing with a doll on the grass. Bammy might be sitting outside with them, crushing mint for her mint sauce, asking Dad to pull her freshly baked rolls from the oven while he made another drink. When we went inside for dinner, we would see out of the corner of our eyes some little Murphy faces peering in our window. Bammy would get up and go to her extra pan of rolls, already split and buttered just for them, and hand them out, along with a jar of her raspberry jam and a spoon.

Mom also invited Dad's folks to dinner. My other grandparents were schoolteachers; Wingie, my grandfather, was now a school principal, and Mammah taught English at a junior high. They loved the world of books, which sat in bookcases with glass covers in their little adobe house on U Street and Second Avenue. Whereas Bammy simply closed her eyes and told stories of her childhood, Mammah would get out a book and read to me. Her special treat was to let me go down the steep, rickety stairs in their musty basement to the grab bag. The grab bag was a pillowcase filled with odds and ends that nowadays would have been tossed in a box for the Goodwill. But Mammah kept every seemingly useless item: an empty thread spool, a lone pretty button, a piece of fabric wrapped in a rubber band, an old-fashioned clothespin. She knew that if you asked a child to close her eyes and reach in and grab three things, but only three, the mysteries of treasure not seen but just felt would hold magic for the whole afternoon. After feeling carefully around in the grab bag, I would come out with three items, and then Mammah and I would plan together what possibilities they held for us. A thread spool became a chair for a fairy; an empty perfume bottle could start a cosmetic counter where I sold many elegant scents; the fabric could be used to wrap and dress a clothespin doll. Mammah never spent money she didn't need to. This drove my father crazy, as by now the Depression was over and life was not so hard. But Mammah and Wingie still persisted in wrapping the dinner rolls from a restaurant and putting them in her purse for breakfast. My father felt it was humiliating.

And even worse than their penny-pinching was their habit of not keeping up with the times. It was a full two years before Wingie realized that the moving pictures were now, some of them, in Technicolor, a phenomenon he proudly announced one night at dinner. My father asked him where he had been for the past couple of years. "Just running the school, son," Wingie said, frowning at my father.

Dad was used to Wingie's frowning. Dad's older brother had enlisted in the navy to fight the Germans and the Japanese, but when Dad went to enlist, he was turned down. His hearing had been damaged through repeated ear infections as a child, in the years before sulfa or penicillin. He was pronounced 4-F, meaning he could not join up to fight. It was the best thing that could have happened for my mother and me, but Dad knew his father was disappointed and he always wanted to do more for the war effort, so instead, he concentrated on his career. He had been a radio announcer and couldn't stand to read aloud all the terrible ads that the producer placed at his microphone. He knew he could write much better ads himself, so in 1938 he had started the R. T. Harris Advertising Agency. It went on to become Harris and Love, one of the most respected ad agencies in the West.

One of Dad's clients was Saltair, our glorious amusement park with a fantastic Moorish dance pavilion set above the lapping waters of Great Salt Lake. It boasted the biggest outdoor dance floor in the world. Louis Armstrong, Harry James, *all* the big bands came to play at Saltair in the early forties, during the war.

One Saturday night back in 1942, four years before Irene was born, it was Dad's job to meet the Glenn Miller Band at the railroad station and send them on a bus out to Saltair, where they'd be playing later that night. Mom was cooking roast beef for

Mammah and Wingie. I, at age three, was running around both-ering everyone. "Take her with you, please," Mom said to Dad, as he started out the door. "I'll give your parents a drink when they come."

So Dad took me along. When Glenn Miller himself stepped off the train, my father ran up and introduced himself. "It is such an honor for me to shake your hand," he said.

Mr. Miller thanked him, organized his band onto the bus, and then turned to Dad and said, "I don't have to be with them as they set up, and I'm just dying for a home-cooked meal. You wouldn't know where there is one nearby, would you? This life on the road can get rough."

Dad told him that Mom was just taking roast beef out of the oven, and would he do us the honor of joining us? Mr. Miller was delighted, and held me on his lap on the way home. This was my first and favorite brush with the famous.

When they got home, Mammah and Wingie were already there, seated around the fire. "Mom and Dad," my father said proudly, "I'd like you to meet Glenn Miller." Dad said it in the same tone as you'd say, "I'd like you to meet . . . God."

My grandfather stood to shake hands. Drink orders were given, and Dad started into the kitchen to help Mom when he heard Wingie say, "What do you do, Mr. Miller?"

My father froze.

"I lead a band," Mr. Miller said cheerfully.

There was a little silence. Mammah said, "Well, that sounds like fun."

Then Wingie said, "Yes, but I meant what do you do for a living?"

Even with his bad hearing, Dad heard that and almost dropped the cocktail tray. Miller was at the height of his career, probably the most famous band leader in the country that year. But Glenn Miller responded kindly and with a twinkle. Dad rushed out to try to educate Wingie, but Mr. Miller just laughed and said, "Actually, I'm trying to join the army." (He would go on to entertain the troops in bases all over Europe, and even arranged a jazzy march for our troops, to the tune of the "St. Louis Blues.")

Wingie brightened and said joining the army and being a soldier seemed like a much more worthwhile job for a fellow, and Dad and the "band leader" burst out laughing.

My father told the story for years. Our household held a lot of hope and laughter then. Irene would come along three years later. Then there was still hope and laughter, but the hope took a different form and the laughter was always a little more uncertain.

2

I Try to Confess

We were not in the habit of praying at our house, although I had been taught "Now I lay me down to sleep." Even though both my parents came from Mormon pioneer stock, over the years they had fallen away from its theology and traditions. Although they had stopped going to church, they sent me anyway. My parents didn't want me to be left out, since they had loved going to church as children. When the teetotaling Mormon home teachers came around to entice them back into the fold, Dad would say, "No, but may I offer you a drink with me? No? Well, then. Come by anytime. Nice to see you. What? Kneel and pray with you? No. No indeed. But how about a nice Manhattan? No? Well, another time then. . . ." He always smiled happily as he showed them out. "Oh, Dick," Mother would say, shaking her head in disapproval and laughing at the same time.

I often invited Mary Frances Murphy to come to our church, because we had lots of activities to which anyone was invited:

talent shows, campouts, taffy-pulling parties. Her parents always shook their heads "no" whenever I asked if she could join me.

It made me wonder why, and what went on in their church that could be more fun. I began to long to go with them, just to see for myself.

All the Murphys went to confession on Saturday evenings. One Saturday I asked if I could go with them. Mrs. Murphy smiled and said she didn't see why not. The sight of the magnificent Cathedral of the Madeleine, hushed and yet filled with mysterious echoes, the fragrance of incense, the jewel tones of the stained-glass windows glowing with the setting sun, simply enchanted me. I watched Mrs. Murphy walk forward to a pew, kneel for just a moment, then get back up and go into the pew, where she promptly knelt again. She took out a beautiful, long string of small pearls, each separated by golden chain. Kneeling and holding the beads, she fingered them and began whispering a prayer. I wondered if she was doing magic. Mr. Murphy went into a wooden box the size of a phone booth and closed the door.

"What's he doing?" I asked Mary Frances.

"He's confessing."

"Confessing what?"

"Well, anything bad he did this week or last week."

"Who does he confess to?"

"A priest."

"And does the priest get mad at him?"

"No, the priest tells him how many prayers he has to say. Then it's all right again because God will forgive him."

I thought about this. I tried to think of a really bad thing I had done, and I couldn't. This was a problem, because I really wanted to see what was in the little box.

I sat in the pew, hearing the footsteps of devout Catholics echo as they walked toward the altar, and I examined my life so far. There must be *something* bad I had done. I closed my eyes and went over any potential sins I could have committed.

Then it hit me: I had done something really rotten that I had buried deep inside myself.

ONCE, WHEN MOM and Dad were having their cocktails by the fire, my baby sister Irene had lost her bottle in her crib and was crying. Mom asked me to run upstairs and give it back to her.

Annoyed at having to go upstairs, I stomped up, went into our bedroom to Irene's crib, found the bottle, and jammed it into her mouth. It wasn't a damaging jolt, but it was hostile enough that it made her start to cry all over again in outrage.

Bammy heard the difference in the cry and came running upstairs. She picked Irene up and cuddled her. "What happened?" she asked, looking at me.

"I have no idea," I said, trying to look innocent.

Bammy frowned at me. She got the bottle, settled Irene in her arms, and started singing, "From this valley they say you are going . . ."

"The Red River Valley" wafted from our little bedroom the way it had when I was a baby, and Bammy's arms made everything cozy and safe again. Irene was asleep in ten minutes.

Sitting there in the pew, I realized that this had been a terrible sin. I'd ask Mrs. Murphy if I could confess as soon as she came past my pew on her way to the confession box.

It had occurred to me that maybe by shoving that bottle

against Irene's little face, I had been the one to damage her brain, and her being slow was all my fault. We knew Mom had trouble having babies because of her arthritis. Why had I come out strong and normal, then? What if Irene had really come out normal too, but my own brutality with that bottle had been the cause of her injury?

By the time Mrs. Murphy came past, I was a puddle of remorse and anxiety.

"Mrs. Murphy!" I whispered loudly.

She turned. "Yes, Terrell?"

"I want to confess!"

She smiled at me. "You can't, honey. You're not Catholic."

Well, this was the worst news of my week. How could I tell God what I had done and ask him to forgive me? How many prayers did I need to learn? Can you really make up for a sin that terrible? Why didn't Mormons get to go confess in a little box every week and have someone forgive them?

When we got home, I announced to my parents that I wanted to be a Catholic.

"Why?"

"I like their beads and their stained glass and their tiny little white prayer books, and it's quiet in their church, not like our church. The Mormons are just so noisy!" I couldn't tell them I just wanted to go into a confession box, to see what it was like, and to be forgiven.

They smiled and looked at each other. Dad said, "You have to wait until you're older. Then you can do anything you want about church."

Gradually, my fascination with confessing subsided, but I

harbored a faint suspicion for years that perhaps I had at least contributed to Irene's disability, if not actually caused it.

Catherine Murphy continued to have lots of babies and look longingly at Mom and her life. She had no idea that Mom's second child would take as much effort as all eight of the children she eventually had.

And of course, neither did we. To this day, our home movies show flickering black-and-white footage of Dad galloping through the living room with Irene on his shoulders; Mom in the kitchen making her famous, fluffy coconut cake or the delicious vinegar chocolate cake; Bammy weeding the Victory Garden and shooing Dad away, shielding her face because she did not look her best for a camera; Dad and me on a sled on a winter morning, scooting down J Street. Every Christmas Eve Dad filmed Irene and me in our pajamas, hamming for the camera, hanging our stockings on the mantel. The stockings we hung were our actual little socks. We did not have giant felt receptacles ready to receive the hundreds of small treasures Americans now feel are necessary. We were thrilled to get some candy, a few small trinkets, and a tangerine in the toe. We looked like a picture-perfect family, right out of *Father Knows Best,* only with a grandmother in the cast. And it felt like one to me. Cozy. Content. Protected. Loved.

You never saw in the home movies that my parents were terrified about Irene. I never saw it, back then, day to day. So it was a complete surprise to me the day Dad turned on me out of the blue.

Irene was two and I was eight. She was sitting on the toilet on her little potty seat with the duck in front. She looked so sweet and sort of helpless, perched on that potty seat. I went into the bathroom and sat down on the edge of the bathtub across from her. I smiled at her and took her little wrists in mine. "Irene," I said, "you are my little sister. Do you know what that means? It means I will always take care of you and I will always protect you." I looked deep into her crossed dark brown velvet eyes, and tears of love welled up in me.

Dad, passing the bathroom, came in. Grabbing my wrists, he said, "What are you doing? Are you twisting her wrists? You leave her alone! She can't defend herself!"

I stared at my father, stunned. Then I got up and ran out of the house.

I leaned against the willow tree, crying at the monstrous injustice done to me. I sobbed and buried my head in the black, wounded, splintered trunk, holding onto it for support. When I had sobbed enough to feel better, I felt that splintered trunk in my hand and realized that it could be a handle. I looked below me and saw another place that could be a foothold. Looking up into the tree, I saw a perfect way to climb into its branches, and hoisted myself up. A thick branch made a perfect seat, and behind it, a backrest for me. I had found my own spot, a place where I could bring my books, hidden from everyone, including my father, who had been mean to me for the first time in my life.

He was my best buddy. I was his pride and joy. He told me so regularly. How could he turn on me like that? I was heartbroken. But up here in my tree, I could escape to my own special place and watch the world go by. I spent every summer for the next four years up in that willow tree when I wasn't playing with friends.

By now Irene was wearing glasses to help straighten her eyes.

Her attention span for any plaything was less than a minute, and then she'd be off wandering again. She squirmed and got up to leave after one page of a storybook. She was sweet, not destructive, just demanding of your attention at all times.

"Mommy? Mommy?"

"What, darling?"

Long silence. Then, "Mommy?" She was trying to form thoughts, but couldn't complete them. When Mom would go on with her tasks, the whole scene would begin again. It was very wearing on everyone.

Irene hung around the house and the backyard, asking her endless, repetitive questions and Bammy and Mom took turns tending her. Irene's attention span was so short that she moved from coloring book to sandpile to swing to dolls, all in the space of five minutes.

Now and then Mammah tried to take Irene for an afternoon, but you could tell that when the few hours were over, she was worn out. "It takes a very patient person to do this," she told Mom. This angered Mom, even though she knew it was true. "Did you hear what she said to me? She actually said Irene is too hard for her to take care of! Of all the nerve! How dare she say that to me!"

Mom was in denial, but, in a way, I sort of understood, because that protective anger rose up in me all though my childhood. When Irene and I were in the backyard with the Murphys, I expected them to be kind to her. I knew how very vulnerable she was, with her little eyeglasses, trying so hard to understand what games we were playing. As we all know, kindness is not in young children's nature. It's not that they're really mean; they just haven't learned to tiptoe around sensitive situations.

Tommy Murphy had a friend, whom I always thought of as Mean Merrill Hall. He once dug up a doll the Murphy girls and I had buried. We'd held a grand funeral for her, too. So when he proudly showed us the shoebox, caked with dirt, we chased him with such fury we actually scared him. Who would rob a doll grave? This guy was evil.

Later, another day, Merrill asked me, "Hey, what's wrong with your sister?" I clenched my fist and tried to punch him in the face. He ducked and backed away.

"Nothing!" I yelled at him. "What's wrong with *you*?" and I lunged for him again. He warded off my blows and ran away.

I'm still looking for him.

The summer I was nine, I came down from my perch in the tree and began to straddle the fence in front of our house instead. I had read every book about horses I could get my hands on, and the fence became my stable. With black crayon, I inscribed the names of my various mounts: Sparky, Silver, Black Beauty, Golden Sovereign. There was one that I had seen in a horse show catalog, Maple Sylvia, only I hadn't grasped the name and wrote "Maple Saliva" instead. Mother had inquired about all this graffiti, but when she saw the pile of library books with the same titles, she understood. "Honey, I am sure you would love a horse. I know you've asked Santa for one for the past three years. It's just that we have no place to keep one! But I'll tell you what we *can* do: we can give you riding lessons at the Wasatch Riding Academy. I'll find out about it. I'll bet you'd make a fine rider."

So every Saturday of that summer and the next, Mom drove me out to the foothills, where I mounted various horses under the tutelage of portly Aunt Sally Benson, who wore false eyelashes and a glittery fringed vest every day we rode. She was also the head of the Gene Autry Riding Club. While Mom sat in the car under a tree and read a novel, I learned to trot, then gallop, then stay on at a flat-out run over those hills. I had a marvelous time.

The winter of 1948 buried Salt Lake City. The snow was almost waist-deep, and the hungry deer strolled out of the mountains and into everyone's backyards. Our Christmas tree glittered in our bay window. On one of the branches was a pair of shoelaces, a family tradition started by Mammah when Dad was just five years old. He had written a note to Santa, saying that he really needed shoes with shoelaces for Christmas. When Mammah asked him about it, he said, "I only have shoes with buckles and I don't know how to tie a bow." Santa brought the laces, and the laces only (after all, he could learn to tie a bow without the extra pair of shoes!). Each year after that, the laces went on the family tree as a poignant symbol of a little boy's need to learn.

Every Christmastime, Dad showed us his home movies, with cartoons and Christmas shows flickering in black and white. My favorite one featured Santa playing sandman, waving sparkling dust over the children's sleeping eyes, then leaving glittering presents under the family's tree before he escaped back up the chimney. I fell asleep dreaming of that movie. In the middle of the night on this wintry Christmas Eve, I woke up and looked out our bedroom window. There, grazing, was the horse Santa must have finally realized I needed so much! I almost wept with joy and ran in to wake my parents.

They staggered in, rubbing their eyes, and peered out the window with me. "Oh honey," my dad said, putting his arm around me. "See, it isn't a horse. It's a deer. A female deer. She sure does look kind of like a horse when she's eating my bushes, doesn't she?"

And then he hugged me, and told me he knew exactly how I felt, because all his childhood he had wanted a bicycle for Christmas, and Santa never thought to bring him one. "But you know what?" he asked, crouching down by me, "that never spoiled Christmas for me. In fact, it made it even more fun, thinking about all the surprises that might be waiting for me. See what I mean?"

For Dad Christmas was all about anticipation: the fun of decorating the tree, the store windows, "Jingle Bells," the endless possibilities of wishes coming true. If they didn't, never mind—the fun was getting ready for it all. He learned to lower his expectations for the things Santa could bring him, and enjoy the season. Every year on June 25, he would announce to us all, "Exactly six months to go! We'd better start planning!"

I told Dad, "I think you should have gotten a bike and I should have gotten a horse."

He laughed. "So do I, honey, so do I, but sometimes life just gives us things to dream about. And guess what! When I was fourteen I earned enough money to get my own bike, so dreams can come true. You just have to make them happen."

"It seems to me, Daddy, that all you ever got for Christmas was a pair of shoelaces, and you had to earn everything else."

He said, "That's about right. But look what it did for me. And I think I love Christmas more than anybody else does."

That summer I learned to ride a bike. I wanted one of my own. One day toward fall I sat with Dad in the vegetable garden, among the warm tomatoes, biting into their juicy red flesh. Dad always brought the sugar bowl along—he liked to sprinkle each bite. It was a little ritual we had together. I asked him, "So Daddy, did you love your bike that you earned?"

"Oh yes, I loved it, for the whole day that I had it."

"You had it only one day? What happened?"

"I rode it to the Pantages Theater to see a movie. It never occurred to me that someone would be so mean as to steal it. But when I came out, it was gone. That was the day I learned the world was not as friendly a place as I thought."

"Did you earn another bike?"

"No, by then I realized I didn't balance very well, because my ears were so bad. I had fallen down so much in one day, riding that bike, it didn't matter that much to me anymore. I would probably have really hurt myself if I'd kept it."

We sat in the sunshine and feasted on our tomatoes. "Maybe one day," I said, "I will get a job and earn a horse. Now I need a horse *and* a bike."

"You show me how you can ride your friend Stephanie's bike and I'll buy you one. As to the horse, that takes a lot of time and money and a stable to keep him in. If you want a horse when you're older, I bet you will earn one."

I put it on my to-do list.

When Gene Autry actually came to town, we riders from Aunt Sally Benson's Gene Autry Riding Club were invited to his suite at the Hotel Utah. When we were ushered into his presence, I gazed upon my first hotel luxury: a big basket of fresh fruit, all wrapped in cellophane and tied with a huge red bow. I was in awe: this is what you get when you're famous.

The Gene Autry Riding Club always rode in the big Twenty-fourth of July parade down Main Street, celebrating the arrival of the Mormon pioneers into Salt Lake Valley. I could hardly wait to be a part of it. That summer I was only ten, and the rule was that you could only ride a horse in the parade if you were twelve years old or over. So the younger riders had to be pioneers on a float that followed the horses and riders.

I was dismayed. My friend in the club, Sheryl Gardner, who was twelve, got to ride a beautiful chestnut horse, and I had to sit on the float in my pioneer dress. I tried to be a good sport about staying with the other younger kids on the float. In our bonnets, full skirts, and aprons, or farmer's hats and pants with suspenders for the boys, we waved to the crowds lining the street, all of us seething inside that we couldn't show off our riding skills from atop horses, where we belonged. I waved to Mom and Dad and Bammy and Irene as they sat on chairs along the street. Irene looked awestruck at the whole idea of the parade. Well, at three years old, a kid is easily impressed, I thought. She has no idea that I am stuck here on this dumb float watching Sheryl Gardner ahead of me on her fancy shiny horse. Sheryl had on a turquoise cowboy hat and a sequined shirt. I could have killed her, I was so envious.

Years later, I met her at a party and told her of that day and my feelings of deprivation and envy.

"Yes," she laughed, "and I was looking at the girl ahead of me on a palomino, all white and shimmery, and I was so envious of her. I wanted to be on the palomino!"

ONE DAY WHEN I was twelve and Irene six, Dad came home with the fanciest gizmo we'd ever seen. The year before, they'd bought an automatic dishwasher, which we all thought was the height of progress. But *this* box held the biggest change ever to happen in our lives at home. It was a television set.

When Dad hooked it up, on came *Kukla, Fran and Ollie,* the puppet show. Irene and I were simply mesmerized. Every day after school, we turned it on, this little black-and-white screen, and the two of us watched it together, our own little ritual. On Saturday nights the whole family gathered around to watch *Your Show of Shows* with Sid Caesar. We were maybe the first on our block to get a set, and Dad was excited about the prospects of advertising in this new medium.

I had been turned out as a commercial actress by my father at the age of three. One of his best clients was Morning Milk, a subsidiary of the Carnation Milk Company in Los Angeles. In an effort to expand their market, Dad thought it would be great if people could be convinced to drink Morning Milk, which was canned and evaporated, instead of just using it for cooking. He needed to show a little kid using it on her cereal, and I was handy. Dad was filming it himself in our dining room. Home movies had only recently been invented, and he had bought one of the first cameras. He set up lights, put the cereal in front of me, checked my dress and hair (Bammy made all my clothes, and I believe I was in fluffy organdy), and rolled the film. This was several years before television, so I wonder now what he was doing filming me. Maybe he had an idea of what was to come, and would show this to his clients as the next way to advertise. "Okay, honey," he said, "now pour the milk on the cereal. No, turn the can so we can see the name on it! That's good. Now pour your sugar on. Keep smiling! Look at the camera and smile again! Good! Now taste your cereal!"

I did exactly what he said. But the cereal with evaporated milk made me wrinkle my whole face up and look for a place to spit it out.

This was a blow to my father. He said that he didn't actually *care* how the cereal tasted with Morning Milk on it; that we would keep doing it again and again until I tasted that stuff with a *happy smile on my face.*

Realizing what might be in store for me for the next hour, I did the whole thing on the second take, and, boy, did I smile! Dad was thrilled. I learned to do things on first takes so I could get on with my life.

It took nine years for Dad's vision of television advertising to come into being. I was already his trained professional. In 1952, every ad was broadcast live. Dad's client, a grocery store chain, advertised every Sunday evening. Dad and I would go to the television station, I would be given my directions, and we would perform little one-minute ads.

You would see my hands putting food in ovens, or in refrigerators. Or you'd see me as the young girl shopping at the store, exchanging dialogue with the fellow who played the store proprietor. Bammy was very proud that I was doing this. "Our Terrell is on television, you know," she'd brag to her bridge group. She never mentioned what I actually *did* on television.

When Bammy and my mother went out for their bridge luncheons, they hired a sweet older woman, Mrs. Grayson, to tend Irene. I would arrive home from school around four o'clock and find Irene and Mrs. Grayson there. Mom hardly ever asked me to relieve the babysitter: she wanted to pay her when she got home, and give me time to myself. I would make myself a sand-

wich of Wonder Bread, butter, and sugar, and curl up happily
with a book on my mom's chaise longue in their bedroom.

It was an afternoon in late spring when Mrs. Grayson came
in to me, looking frightened, but saying calmly, "Terrell, something is very wrong with me. I need you to call an ambulance.
Tell them to come here right away."

Holding her head with both hands, she went into our bathroom and closed the door. I could hear her moaning and crying.
My heart pounding, I picked up the phone to call the emergency
number. Someone was on our party line, chatting away. "Excuse
me," I said, "this is an emergency. Could you please hang up
while I call for an ambulance?"

"How old are you, dear?"

"Twelve. Please. I really need to get help here."

"You kids are all alike. The minute you want to use the phone,
you try to get us to hang up."

"Please. This is not a joke, honest! Our babysitter is in the
bathroom and I think she may be dying!"

"If you're twelve, what are you doing with a babysitter, huh?"

"Oh, please! Please! Help me!"

Finally, they gave in and hung up.

I got the ambulance people, gave them the address, and then
called Dad. "I'm on my way. Good girl." I went into the bathroom then to see if I could do anything for Mrs. Grayson. She
had been sitting on the toilet, but had collapsed and fallen off.
She was wedged in between the sink and the toilet, and blood
was pouring out of her nose and mouth onto the white tile.

Irene was standing in the hall, both hands in her mouth,
her eyes wide in horror. We heard the sirens wailing as they

approached our house. Doors slammed and the paramedics ran up the stairs.

Just then Dad arrived home, followed by Mrs. Grayson's daughter, who was also terrified, and crying, "Oh no! Oh no!" as she watched her mother being carried out on the stretcher. The ambulance people had already called for a hearse, which arrived shortly afterward. Dad said, "Terrell, you and Irene go stand outside under the willow tree, so that when Mom and Bammy drive in, they'll see you two are okay."

We did. Irene watched as Mrs. Grayson's body was transferred from the ambulance to the hearse, her daughter weeping and following. Mrs. Grayson had died of a massive brain hemorrhage.

Irene stayed quiet, but inside she was not calm. To this day, she still frets over ambulance sirens, asking constant questions about who is hurt, are they dying? The next day she will still be worried about it. As for me, there are still times when I go into a ladies' room and open a stall door, and for just a brief moment I see Mrs. Grayson lying there.

3

We Find Out the Truth

The sadness of Mrs. Grayson's death began our year of bad news and change. Irene entered kindergarten in September 1951, and that's when we found out how injured her brain really was. After the very first day, the teacher telephoned and asked my parents to come and see her the next day after school.

She told them that Irene was unable to do most of the things her fellow classmates could, and she suggested they have Irene tested at the University of Utah. She sent them to a well-respected professional in the field of special education.

When the test results came back, the professor gave them this news:

1. Your child is mentally disabled with an IQ of around 57.
2. She will never learn to read and write.
3. She will make lots of friends and she responds well to loving attention.
4. Her emotional age is around three, which means she will

not have the emotional capacity to empathize with others. Ever.

5. Her explosive temper outbursts are not because she is spoiled. This is very common to this population: their brain chemistry wires them for tantrums.

6. Although she responds to love and affection and has some social skills, she will probably never marry because her emotional skills are not up to that.

7. She does not fit into normal public schools. There are no programs where she would fit in, except, of course, at the state institution. Many parents have chosen this option.

8. So sorry.

WHAT HAD CAUSED Irene's brain damage? Looking back on her difficult birth, her crossed eyes, her delayed reactions and abnormal behaviors, the professor concluded that she was a victim of anoxia, or lack of oxygen to the brain, during her birth. There was no going back and making it right. Mom probably should have had a cesarean, but she'd had a substitute doctor that day, and in his judgment, it hadn't been necessary.

Bammy never forgave that doctor for putting my mother through that labor and delivery when he could have used safer methods. Now and then she would shake her head and say, "He will pay for that sin, just you watch. If not now, he will in heaven." Then her eyes would narrow and she would add, "If he gets to heaven at all."

Mom and Dad went over it again and again in their minds, and finally realized they had to move on and decide what to do now.

In the opinion of most Americans of that time, it was best to send these children away, so that they could "be with their own kind." Either that, or keep them out of sight of the rest of the neighborhood. It was too unpleasant, you see.

So my parents went down to take a look at our state institution in American Fork, about sixty miles south of Salt Lake City. They saw large, smelly rooms of children and adults, all with some handicap or other, some engaged in an activity, others staring blankly or longingly out the window. They couldn't bear the thought of leaving her there.

They came home and said that Irene was not going to the state training school.

Bammy was making her delicious swiss steak, handed down from her pioneer mother. She listened carefully to them, frowning the whole time. "I don't want people making fun of her," she said as she slathered mustard over the meat. "Children can be so cruel." She piled slices of onions and then fresh tomatoes from the garden onto the steak. "If you keep her home, she's staying right inside the house with me." She sprinkled a bit of sugar over the tomatoes and put the pan in the oven.

Mom watched her thoughtfully, worried that Bammy was ashamed of her little namesake. But that wasn't the case.

What Bammy didn't tell us then, what she never told any of us, was something I found out about half a century later.

Bammy, who had been born in 1899 to a prominent pioneer family, had had a half-brother who was mentally retarded. Her mother had kept George in a little house of his own, behind the family house. He was never allowed out in company, or with the family either. A helper always looked after him, and it was agreed that no one would ever mention him. One grainy family photo, I am told, shows the whole family on a picnic, and one child in a cage. It must have been George. Her father had been the mayor, and George was his son by his second wife in polygamy, who had died. In Salt Lake City in the late 1800s, you would never admit to the community that you had a child that "wasn't right." It was a sign of weakness.

With this news, Mom said we had to move into a bigger house, with more than one bathroom and a separate bedroom for Irene. I would be entering junior high. Mom knew I'd be having homework and telephone calls, and sharing a bedroom just wouldn't work anymore. She thought I would be happy.

She was wrong. I was devastated. I didn't mind sharing a room with Irene, and I loved our little house and my willow tree and my fence that turned into horses for me. I loved the neighborhood kids, Tommy Murphy and Mean Merrill Hall notwithstanding. I did not want my childhood to end. But Dad painted over the horses' names on the fence in front and spruced up the house for sale. I was heartbroken. Dad took me for a ride in the car and talked to me about it. "Honey, I can see this looks like an end of happy times to you. But we have to do this. Our house is just too small. Could you think of this as the beginning of new and wonderful times?"

I could not. My happy, secure childhood in my little gabled bedroom was over. Mom and Dad's ribbon and roses wallpaper was over. My life as a sidekick to the Murphy family was over. Who would be my friends and neighbors now?

Mom and Dad bought a big old house in Federal Heights, at 1383 East South Temple. Bammy said, "You know, this is a much more fashionable part of town." She was all for improving one's station in life.

I hated it. I hated a big house. I wanted a cozy little house. When it came time for us to leave 518 J Street, I remember praying, "Please let me come back here. Please. I'll do anything to earn it. Just let me know. I'll do it. This is my real home. No other house will be home to me, ever." As we drove away, I looked back longingly at the Murphys' house, and Tenth Avenue, and all I loved as warm and familiar.

God was silent on the matter.

My notion that we had moved into a strange house was proven when Bammy set up her iron and ironing board in the large upstairs hall. When she plugged in the iron, the doorbell rang nonstop for five minutes and then stopped. Dad inspected the wiring, and when he couldn't fix it, he called electricians, who couldn't fix it either. For all the years we lived in that house, we knew when Bammy was ironing because the doorbell would ring endlessly. We learned to ignore it.

But a few days after we moved to the new house, I got even more of a surprise. It was about eleven at night, and everyone was, I thought, asleep in bed. I was looking for my hairbrush, which I'd left in Irene's room. I knew Irene was never bothered by lights being on after she was asleep, so I flipped the switch so I could see.

My father was kneeling at her bedside. His forehead was resting on his folded hands. I could not even imagine it. I believe he was praying.

At the shock of the light going on, he rose quickly and whispered, "Don't you *ever* turn a light on like that again!"

Irene slept blissfully through this scene, but my pain was already so great at losing my childhood home and my willow tree that Dad's anger left me doubled up in my bed, weeping, my head and heart protected under my covers.

Looking back on it now, I am sure that he was embarrassed that I found him on his knees, so vulnerable, asking for help.

He'd never admit it, but I think his answer came very quietly. Because only a few days later, Dad took action.

4

Childhood's End

Letter to the Editor, *Salt Lake Tribune*, September 1952

> I am a parent of a mentally retarded girl, six years old. I
> plan to keep her at home, but I want her to learn as much
> as she is capable of learning. I find there are no programs
> for her in the Salt Lake Valley. If you are a parent with a
> similar problem, and would like to form a group to begin
> a day care center, please call me at 35644.
>
> *Richmond T. Harris*

Most days that first September of junior high, I would come
home from school to a babysitter tending Irene, as Mom and Bam
were often off to their lunch and bridge games. The phone would
be ringing off the hook.

"Hello? Is this the home of Mr. Harris?"

"Yes," I would answer, pulling out the big pad of paper
where I was keeping names and phone numbers.

"My child is mentally retarded. I have never said this to anyone before." Then the sobbing would begin. I would wait until it subsided, and then I would say, "My dad wants me to take down your name and phone number, and he'll call you back tonight. They're going to have a meeting. He wants you to come."

"Oh, bless you, my child. Thank God someone had the courage to put it out there in the paper!"

By the time my father called the meeting, he had fifty names.

They met at the State Capitol Building. When they finished telling their stories to each other, they cried, they laughed, and they hugged each other in the relief of finding others in the same boat. They resolved to pool their money, find some space to rent, hire a teacher, and open a day care center. They organized into the Salt Lake County Association for Retarded Children. Within a few weeks, they had rented a small, rundown, vacant clubhouse on the grounds of Fairmont Park. On Saturday mornings, everyone pitched in to clean it up, paint it, and get it ready for their children. All the families helped, including brothers and sisters. I remember sweeping the floor while Dad measured spaces for worktables. Mothers and sisters washed the windows. Irene and the other children who would attend the center played outside in the park.

We didn't know that simultaneously, all over the country, day care centers were being created by other parents of children with mental disabilities. In fact, other states had a two-year jump on us. In 1950, forty people from thirteen states, all of them veterans of opening day care centers in their own towns, had already met in Minneapolis and formed the National Association for Retarded Children. They felt that it was time to "stop agonizing and start organizing." What they accomplished is the stuff of legend.

If Irene would never read, so be it; but my parents would never give up helping her to be the best that she could be. And at last, she had somewhere to go every day, as other children did. She could meet new friends and learn new skills. She would have a happy life in the community.

Thanks but No Thanks

Okay, here's one: A man goes to get a taxicab, and he sees this poor heavy woman struggling in the door of the cab. She is so obese that she is stuck, with her back out the door. He puts his hand on her back to help her, and with all his strength he finally succeeds in getting her into the cab, whereupon she turns around, reaches out the window, and hits him with her purse.

"But madam," he says, "I was trying to help you get in!"

"In!" she yells. "I was trying to get out!"

And this is how it was with advocacy for mentally handicapped kids. Even with all Dad's efforts to get things going for these children, a lot of them didn't want to leave the house after all. Irene was one of the homebodies. Life was good at home. Our mother and grandmother waited on her, giving her constant attention. What was not to like? To show us how much she wanted to stay home, she threw tantrums. Down-on-the-floor, screaming, legs-kicking tantrums.

Every morning, Mom and Bammy would wrestle Irene into her clothes as she yelled that she didn't want to go. Then they would bundle her into the car, and Dad would drive her to the day care center while she screamed, kicked the windshield, and socked her own face until her nose bled. He tried everything:

threats, bribery, spanking, you name it. Didn't work. It took all he had every morning to get her to go in the door of the center. It was only after she was inside and realized Dad was leaving and she was there for the day that she gave up and calmed down.

I didn't have to go through this horror every morning. I had my own horror: adolescence. Hello twelve, hello thirteen, hello boys, hello boobs, hello pimples. Also hello being taller than every boy in the whole world of seventh grade. Our mothers, in an effort to help us all out, enrolled many of us in the neighborhood in Arthur Murray dance classes, held once a month at the Center for the Blind. There we learned the art of the box step, tentatively holding on to each other, not daring to look each other in the eye. We stared fixedly at our feet as we box-stepped around the room. It was a good thing that we all looked down. If the boy stared straight ahead, he would be looking at my breasts, which would have embarrassed him as much as me. My chest was bigger than most of my friends', and I despised it.

My spirits picked up when they taught us how to do the swing. Our parents called it the jitterbug, and were delighted that we were learning it. Slow, slow, quick-quick, slow. By spring several of the boys started to get taller, and were actually looking more at my throat now. This encouraged me no end.

When we had dances at school or the local Mormon ward, I was invited by various boys from the dancing class. The trouble was, any boy who came to my house as a prospective date got to meet my sister. When they walked in the door, Irene would usually be right there, asking them, "Hi, where's your mommy? Wanna talk to my doll?" I was too young to have a sense of humor about it. That came later. At this stage, as with pimples and periods, I chose to close my eyes and get through the experience as quickly as possible, and the boy and I would be out the door and on our way. We just didn't discuss Irene. I was far too insecure.

The only thing that got me through junior high was athletics: first, competitive swimming; then, ice skating. I lived in the swimming pool of the Deseret Gymnasium for about three years, becoming intermountain breaststroke champion at age fourteen. Then I fell madly in love with ice skating. I took the bus to the rink every day after school and skated until Dad picked me up around six o'clock. When I became truly addicted to it, Dad even got up at five in the morning to get me to the rink so I could skate for two hours before school. I had met another friend, Lynne, who skated with me; her mother picked us up after we skated, cooked us breakfast, and drove us to school, where we yawned our way through classes for three more years.

Irene took lessons, too, and learned to both swim and skate, which surprised us all. Her swimming stroke was a dog paddle. On the ice, she didn't want to jump and spin as I did, but she loved her private lessons each week, made it around the rink and learned to skate backward a little bit. She was very proud of it, as were we.

Looking back on my years of living at swimming pools or ice rinks, I suppose a psychologist would say, "Well, you were escaping your home situation with your sister," but that's not how it felt at all. I was truly in love with the sports. "Well, then," says my imaginary shrink, "you were overcompensating for your sister, trying to be so outstanding for your parents, to make up for her lack of abilities."

Could be, I guess. But if that's true, it was surely lost on them. I would come home from a swim meet, driven by another of the swim team's parents, and Mom and Dad would be playing bridge with friends. "Hey, guys, I won the hundred-meter breaststroke in both age divisions," I'd say, putting my trophies on the card table for all to admire. "Honey, that's wonderful!" my parents would say, and then hand me back the trophies because it was on the dummy's hand and they needed to get on with their game. They never saw me swim in a race. It was a far cry from today's overly eager parents at swim meets.

As to skating, one morning on the way to the rink, Dad said, "Listen, hon. I've been thinking. Your swimming used to cost me maybe fifty dollars a year. Add thirty more for the six swimsuits you went through each year. Your skating costs me that almost every week! I have a great idea: go back to the pool! Or, here's an idea: let's think up a new sport—deep breathing! Completely without cost to fathers! What do you say, huh?"

I told him that soon I would have a driver's license and maybe that would help matters. "And you expect to borrow the one car we have?"

"I can drive Irene to her tutoring lessons, think of that."

He looked over at me. "You're going to go far in this world, you know that?"

Meanwhile, Mom was busy trying to get Irene integrated into neighborhood life as well as being in a special school. She became a Brownie leader for a troop of little girls that included Irene. She also taught primary, the Mormon youth group for elementary school children. Irene was a model student in both situations. It was the little boys who gave Mom trouble. One little kid named Peter was causing so many problems while they were constructing Indian teepees that Mom started to cry, startling Peter into dead silence. Rising to her full height, Mom sniffed into her

hanky and said, "Peter, you just take your teepee and go home!"
It became a family saying for whenever we were at our wit's end
with someone.

By the time I got my driver's license, Irene had settled down
somewhat on the tantrums in the car, at least when I drove her to
her reading tutors in the afternoon. My parents never, ever gave
up on trying to get her to read and write. We must have had
twenty different tutors who gave it their all. To this day, Irene
will pass a home or apartment building, point to it, and say,
"'Member I went there for reading lessons?" I had completely
forgotten, but not Irene.

It never worked. Irene can write her name in very large letters,
the way you do in kindergarten, but that's all. She reads her
name on an envelope, but the rest is a mystery to her. She does,
however, recognize symbols and icons from advertising. "There's
Clover Club potato chip's truck! There's my Winder milkman!"
They were all Dad's clients, and he worked hard to get their name
everywhere.

His brilliant work in the advertising business was paying well.
All his life, Dad had wanted to travel, but he could never afford it
until now. He and Mom had gone to Hawaii with friends in 1950,
and though it rained every day, they came home aglow with the
travel bug. Now they wanted to go to Europe. Unbelievably to
me as I look back on it now, they didn't consider just the two of
them going: of course they would take the whole family, including Bammy. It would be an education for us all.

Can you picture floating along a canal in Venice in the moon-
light, the gondolier serenading you? Your arm is around your
dear wife, and across from you is your mother-in-law? And behind her are your two daughters, the little one in glasses wailing

because she thinks the gondola is going to tip over? Apparently my father could.

Bammy didn't much like Europe. When we landed at Orly Airport in Paris, she asked why we had to stand in line with our luggage. "They need to see our passports and make sure we're safe tourists," Dad told her.

"Well, just tell them we're Americans and they'll let us right on through," Bammy assured him. Only seven years earlier, Americans had liberated their country from the Germans, and she expected royal treatment.

Then there was the language. "What are those people saying about us?" she asked suspiciously as the nasal sounds of French wafted around the airport. "The little snips. They just do that to annoy us," she said.

When we checked into the Hôtel Napoléon, she saw her first bidet. "What's that for?"

"To wash your bottom," Mom told us all.

Bammy regarded it with narrowed eyes. "Don't these people have toilet paper?"

When she tried their toilet paper, which at that time felt like sandpaper, she knew she'd had enough of the whole continent. "Well, that's enough now. Let's all go home."

"Bam, we haven't even unpacked. Now let's do that and go have a lovely dinner in a little bistro near here."

When she tasted their beef bourguignon, she muttered, "It's just beef stew, only mine is better."

On the plane to England, I made friends with a lovely older gentleman named Mr. Bristowe. He insisted on taking us all to dinner and showing us around London. At dinner, he peered at us all over his rimless glasses and told us how much he admired our country. I looked over at Irene sitting next to him. She had slipped her glasses down on her nose and was looking at us over them, in the same manner as Mr. Bristowe. My father was afraid Mr. Bristowe would think Irene was making fun of him, but he laughed, patted her head, and made sure she ordered the best pudding for dessert.

When it came, it was cake. "This is cake, not pudding," Bammy said.

"Yes, madame. That is what you call dessert and we call pudding. All our desserts are puddings."

Bammy frowned at him, but didn't say anything until we got back to the hotel. Putting on her nightgown, she muttered, "Pudding. For heaven's sakes. No one speaks English over here."

At Buckingham Palace, Irene went up to one of the guards, who was standing totally immobile, staring straight ahead. Irene stood very close to him and peered up at him. No response. She touched his bright red coat and stared up at his beaver fur hat. She had seen this before at home, under our Christmas tree. A nutcracker! When I approached her to tell her to come along, she was chatting happily at the silent, staring guard. She beamed at me. "This is a dolly?" she asked. She was trying to hold his hand. His mouth twitched, but he kept looking straight ahead.

Bammy insisted on using the iron she brought along because no family member of hers was going to dinner looking wrinkled. She put two different old inns in Ireland completely in the dark for several hours by plugging our iron into their sockets. When she was told our plugs would not work in their wall sockets, she simply huffed, and said, "Well, they should," and went right on with her task. When the second outage occurred, Dad was reading his guidebook by lamplight. Suddenly plunged into the dark, he swore and said to Mom, "Bam's ironing again." This time his phone rang, and it was Bammy from our room, whispering. "Dick! Did I do that?"

"Yes, you did, Bam. We've been trying to tell you." What was it about Bammy and irons?

"Well, how can we go out to dinner in wrinkled dresses?"

In the small Irish towns we were traveling in, there were no converters to be found. No one seemed to notice we were disheveled.

When we finally flew out of Shannon Airport toward New York, Bammy let out a long sigh of relief. "They need to come to our country and taste *real* food," she announced.

Mom and Dad had been thrilled with the whole trip, power outages and all. For our family, it was the adventure of a lifetime. Now it was time to attend to other family needs, most especially, Irene's crossed eyes, which had never straightened by themselves. Irene was now ten and the doctor said it was a good age to get her eye muscles tied surgically. The operation went well. She stumbled around the house with her eyes bandaged for a week. When they took the bandages off, she still wouldn't open her eyes. Then, hours later, at dinner, we watched her slowly blink them open. She looked around at all of us. "Hi!" Dad said to her. She looked at each one of us as if seeing us anew. Maybe she was. "Where my glasses are?" she asked.

"You don't need them anymore, sweetie! Can you see us better?"

"I don't need my glasses?"

"That's right." We were looking closely at her eyes, which indeed were straighter, but not perfect. At least she looked a little more normal, even if she didn't act it.

Neither, for that matter, did I. To most kids, normal was being a cheerleader, not on the staff of the school newspaper. Normal was hanging out together at Farr's Ice Cream Shop, not curled up alone on the couch reading humorists such as Robert Benchley, James Thurber, and S. J. Perelman or the western writer A. B. Guthrie Jr. Normal was going out with football players, not guys on the newspaper staff, all of whom came up to my chin and wore big horn-rimmed glasses. Besides, they were horrid dancers. I wanted Fred Astaire.

As I went from twelve to sixteen, I gained the wisdom and maturity to handle boys and their attitudes toward my sister. Besides, my pimples went away, the boys got taller, and all the other girls got breasts in some measure or another. I was more comfortable in my own skin.

When a boy came to the house now, it was still the same routine with Irene. "Hi! Where's your mommy? Wanna talk to my doll?" If the boy turned away from her and pretended not to hear, I smiled and said she had some special ways of communicating. I would never say, in front of her, that she was brain-damaged. I also would not go out with that boy again.

If he answered her question as if this were par for the course, I'd think he had potential. It must have been a disquieting experience for a boy to cross my threshold, to have to explain where his mommy was, and talk to Irene's favorite, disheveled doll; but some, like handsome, articulate Bob Coles, actually smiled and answered. Bob, who wanted to be a journalist, felt comfortable around us all. Mostly, though, the ones who were nicest to her were the short nerds. They were my pals, but not glamorous material.

After a steady diet of Gene Kelly, Fred Astaire, and Gregory

Peck on the movie screen, I really wanted more. After all, my idol was Esther Williams, and I swam just like her, I thought. I deserved a romantic hero, big and bold and brawny.

After hinting broadly to everyone I knew, I managed at last to convince a cheerleader to take pity on me and line me up with the strong, tall, sexy Marlowe Smith. At last I was going to be squired about by the hunk I knew I deserved. When he picked me up, there was Irene and the rest of my family. My father shook hands with him, Mother and Bammy looked him up and down, and then Irene asked, "Where's your mommy?"

Marlowe flinched. He turned away from them and whispered to me, "What is wrong with her?"

Now of course this was a sure sign that I should dump this loser, but this was the captain of the football team! The only boy in the school taller than me! I would have eloped with him that evening if he'd asked.

More comfortable in my own skin. Wisdom and maturity. Right. Except sometimes.

Smiling and simpering, I said, "Never you mind about my sister, Marlowe. Let's go to the movie," and away we went. I felt completely glamorous. I had a fine time at the movie and, later, being seen with Marlowe by many classmates at the ice-cream store. He wasn't the best conversationalist, but I didn't care. I talked enough for both of us.

As we walked up to my front door at the end of the evening, Marlowe shook my hand very formally, and then said, "Terrell. Can I ask you a question?"

My mind raced. Was he going to ask me out again? The school dance was coming up! My heart was pounding. Or was he going to ask about my little sister?

"Sure, Marlowe! What?"

"How come you use so many big words?"

My heart sank. I thought back on our date. What on earth had I said? Marlowe had muttered only a few words the whole night, most of them one syllable. My glamorous social future was over. "Well, Marlowe, I guess that's just how I am. I am so sorry!"

He shrugged, pulled his East High letter jacket tighter against the winter night, turned on his heel, and left me forever. I was devastated.

For about a week. Then I went back to the short nerds who could speak in long, thoughtful sentences as we put out the school newspaper together. Besides, we were all studying so hard to get good marks for our college applications, I didn't have much time for romantic longing.

Dad had always admired Stanford University, and hoped I'd apply there, so I did. By early spring quarter of my senior year, I got the news. My best friend Jeannie and I would both be going to Stanford.

One day I was asked on a date by Paul Dougan, who had grown up in my neighborhood and was already a sophomore at Stanford. When he walked in the door, Irene was right there with her perennial question. He answered in all sincerity, "Where's my mommy? My mom is just up the street on Fourth Avenue, Irene. We live four blocks away. Would you like to come and meet her?"

Bammy, who was standing in the hall too, said, "Oh my heavens, you're Helen Dougan's boy. Why, I've played bridge at your house many times! I've watched you and your brother since you were babies. I just love your mother. Come right in and have dinner with us."

When Paul took me to our local dance pavilion at Lagoon, and we danced to Louis Armstrong and his band, I found that his box step lacked a certain rhythm. In fact, he stepped on my feet every other beat and seemed to have adopted a sort of whirling step that had a life of its own and made us both completely dizzy. I was about to suggest we go get a lemonade when the Armstrong band broke into a great swing number. Suddenly Paul took my hand and turned into Fred Astaire. "How do you know how to jitterbug?" I asked, full of wonder. "Arthur Murray!" Paul answered. "Slow, slow, quick-quick, slow."

We were soul mates right then and there. He was funny, very smart, loved by all his friends, and best of all, he was six-foot-one.

At Christmas, he showed up at our door with a large gift for me under his arm. It was a big doll, an Emmett Kelly clown, which threw Irene into complete raptures. She held the doll all Christmas Day. "Wow, this thoughtful guy really must be in love with me," I thought to myself. Paul took me to a movie that night, and Callie, the girl in the box office who also worked at the gift shop, handed us our tickets and asked, "Hey, Paul, I loved that clown you bought at the store yesterday. Did you ever decide which of your girlfriends to give it to?"

Paul pointed at me, totally chagrined.

"Okay, Mr. Romance, let's go see the movie," I told him.

We've told this to our daughters more times than they cared to hear it.

5

College and Onward

At East High, I was a reasonably outstanding student. At Stanford, I dog-paddled in a sea of incredibly outstanding students. My three swim trophies were dwarfed by the hundreds of trophies of my fellow students, one of whom was already on the U.S. Olympic Team. My roommates were brilliant. One roommate, Joan, never went to class at all. She never bought a textbook: she just borrowed mine the night before a test, lit a cigarette, thumbed through the book, and got an A the next day. I slaved away in the stacks, trying to absorb all my subjects, and for the first time I sort of knew how Irene must feel around the rest of the world. I never failed a class, and got Bs and Cs, but I felt totally out of my element. And the partying at night simply shocked me. Paul took me to a fraternity party, where two of his frat brothers got roaring drunk and put their fists through all the windows at the hall they'd rented. I was horrified. Besides, it wasn't any fun.

Then we'd go to the Mormon parties, where we'd play

musical chairs in couples, where you sat on the boy's lap as the chairs got pulled away. We played relay games: pass the lifesaver on a toothpick using just your lips. Or pass the orange holding it under your chin, no hands allowed. A marvelous game. No alcohol. Great music. Lots of fun.

I went out with other boys. They seemed on another planet to me, and I must have to them. I was so straight, did not drink, and kept all dorm rules that said I had to be in by eleven, or midnight on weekends. This is what happens when you grow up Mormon in Salt Lake City. We flinched at the thought of overdue library books. We never jaywalked. We followed all the rules. We shared the same history, spoke the same language.

It was Stanford's language that was passing strange. I went to one football game with Paul. At the gate he said, "Well, see you after the game."

"Why after the game? Aren't we sitting together?"

"No. I'm in the card section."

"The card section! Where you hold up cards? I would love to do that! I hate football! Give me a hot dog and put me in the card section and I will be a happy camper!"

"Only men get to work the cards."

Only men got to be in fraternities at Stanford, too, in those years. Plus, they had a motto, those adorable Stanford boys: "Nine out of ten girls are beautiful. The tenth one goes to Stanford." Because they couldn't stand our competing with them in class, the boys tended to date girls from San Jose State. My friend Jeannie came to me in our sophomore year and said, "Let's go home. I hate this place. Paul will be graduating and going into the navy, and then who would you want to go out with anyway?"

She had a point. Besides, our education did not seem any better than what our friends were getting back home. As undergraduates, especially the first two years, it seemed we were getting very few full professors, just teaching assistants. Jeannie wanted to join a sorority and have some fun for just a few minutes. I didn't blame her. Thus we put in for transfers out, to the horror of the Stanford staff. My counselor suggested I take a psychological test to see if I was mentally competent. Anyone who didn't like Stanford must have a screw loose. "Anyway," he said, "it will show you where your skills might lie for a future career."

So I took the test. My highest skill, it said, would be as an elevator operator.

I didn't mind. I had been doing a little work on my own. I was already a college correspondent for *Good Housekeeping,* and I'd entered the *Mademoiselle* magazine College Board contest. If you won, you got to go to New York and guest-edit the magazine with their staff for a month. One of my projects had been a short story. Just after I put it in the mail, my Stanford creative writing teacher called me in to his office for a consultation. "This is a terrible story," he said. "You'll have to do this assignment over. All this shows is the cruelty of children. And then it ends with a funny story."

I was feeling faint. "Well, yes, that's what I meant to show," I said.

"Well, it's stupid. It tries to make you cry and laugh all at the same time. What do you expect the reader to do? Cry or laugh?"

"Well, both. That was my thought," I told him. "I just put it in the mail to the *Mademoiselle* contest."

His eyes got wide, and then narrowed meanly. "If you had the unmitigated gall to submit that to *Mademoiselle,* you really are dumber than I thought."

I felt my eyes well up with tears, and I promised I would write him something else. Spring quarter was almost over, and I had to get a grade from him to transfer to the University of Utah. I stumbled back to the dorm, blinded by tears, wondering what else to write. I had just written of my experiences on Tenth Avenue as a child. I must be a horrible writer and had never known it.

I struggled for two weeks, in between classes and other studies, to write a better story for him. But I liked the one I had written and could not think what would please this man.

Then it arrived. Trembling, I opened Western Union's yellow envelope. "Congratulations. You have been chosen as a 1959 Guest Editor. Please make arrangements to be in New York by June 1. And tell us whom you would like to interview. Sincerely, the staff at *Mademoiselle*."

When I called *Mademoiselle* I got Lisa Hopping, who had been one of the judges. "Oh, Terrell!" she said happily. "I'm so glad you can come."

"Tell me, please, which of my four projects convinced you to choose me?"

"Oh! Your short story, hands down! We're not going to publish it or anything. I really just wanted to meet you. You sound fun. Now, tell me who I can work on getting for you to interview?"

"Would Danny Kaye be too much to ask for?" My father and I worshipped him.

"I'll see what I can do. See you in June!"

Then I went to each of my instructors and arranged to take my finals early, because I had to be in New York before finals week. When I got to my creative writing teacher, he seemed both stunned and furious. I told him time was running out to write him another story, and as a matter of fact, that very story was what had got me to be one of the twenty winners.

"Go!" he said bitterly. "I'll just take that story as your submission to me. Just go!"

And he turned his back on me and stared out the window. I later learned that this man had received an award for his novel manuscript, but could never find anyone who wanted to publish it.

Paul drove me to the airport to fly to New York. "Now how much money do you have in your wallet?" he asked.

I looked. "Twelve dollars." I thought that was quite a bit.

"Oh *that's* good," he laughed, reaching for his wallet. He handed me $60. "You'll have to walk to the hotel unless you take this."

I don't know why I never thought of that. Paul just kept on looking more and more like a fellow you'd want to have around. We hugged good-bye, and I climbed on the plane with another Stanford girl, Geri Wilder, who had also won the contest. We both opened and showed each other our second yellow telegrams. She was going to interview the actor John Houseman. Mine said, "Danny Kaye unavailable. Will James Thurber do?"

Thurber was one of my all-time idols. I had nearly passed out.

That month in New York dazzled all twenty of us guest editors from colleges around the country. We went backstage at *My Fair Lady* and got to try on their elegant hats. We were introduced to all sorts of actors and heads of corporations. The Fieldcrest Company gave us each an invitation that said, "Your transportation to our offices awaits you in the morning in front of your hotel." When we walked out that morning, ten horse-drawn carriages from Central Park were lined up, waiting to transport us down Fifth Avenue. Meeting my idol, James Thurber, gave me goose bumps. He had gone completely blind by this point and was gloomy. He asked what I wanted to be in life. "I'd like to be a homemaker and a writer," I told him.

He said, "Humph. Every housewife has a novel in her apron pocket." I shook his hand and slunk away. Never mind. What he contributed to American humor can never be diminished, and if he was a little grumpy in his old age, I totally forgive him.

We interviewed Samuel Goldwyn in his hotel room at the Sherry-Netherland. I asked him how he came to have the roaring lion as the logo for MGM films. He told us he had taken his daughter to the zoo just as he and his partners were starting up their company, and his daughter had been in awe of the lion that roared. "That's what I wanted people to feel when they saw our films," he said.

On my own I went to eleven shows on Broadway. We stayed at the Barbizon Hotel for Women; they had house rules for young ladies, to be in by eleven on weeknights, midnight on weekends.

It was years before I learned of the famous poet Sylvia Plath and *The Bell Jar.* When I finally read it, I realized she had had the same experiences at *Mademoiselle* just six years before I did. Where she was paralyzed with the choices of career before her, and despondent at the materialism of all the goodie bags we got, I was simply thrilled. They gave us clothing and cosmetics and all sorts of gifts. Apparently this depressed Sylvia so much that she went up on the roof of the Barbizon Hotel and handed all her beautiful new clothes to the wind.

She went on to become one of the most famous, and probably the most tortured, women in American literature. In the midst of her career, with two little babies in their cribs upstairs, she put her head in the oven and killed herself. I thought maybe the most brilliant writers might just be the most unbalanced, but then I realized Joyce Carol Oates had also been a *Mademoiselle* guest editor, so it appears you can indeed be brilliant and lead a satisfying life.

I dated two boys from Salt Lake while in New York. There was so much to do I was almost too excited to sleep, and came home with a galloping case of mononucleosis. Paul came back from a geology field trip to find me bedridden.

He brought dinner over and served it to me like a professional waiter. I felt completely cared for. We couldn't kiss, because of my disease. He didn't care. I put my head on his lap and we watched television after his dinner of steak, baked potatoes, and pecan pie.

Bammy was really impressed. "That," she said, "is a man you can count on."

It seemed so comfortable, and so right, to both of us. Paul told me later he told his mother that he was planning to ask me to marry him, and she thought for a minute and then asked, "Is she healthy?" Looking at our family, with Mom's arthritis, Dad's poor hearing, and Irene's damaged brain, you would have to wonder.

Just before Paul left for his stint in the navy, he took my parents and me to lunch and asked them for my hand in marriage. They hugged him. They knew he was a man of substance and character. He gave me a beautiful diamond, but we put it away until we could see our future, and the best time to announce our engagement. If his navy stint kept him on the ship for two years, I could keep the diamond in my drawer, go to parties with friends, and finish college. But he thought his duty would not be on a ship. He would let me know the minute he found out.

My friend Jeannie and I had felt we were missing out on fun at Stanford, and sorority life appealed to us. We went through rush at the university and each pledged different sororities. Jeannie thought it was all quite wonderful.

It turned out I absolutely hated it. Sorority life as a junior, after the rigors of Stanford study, left me feeling just as alienated as I had on campus at Stanford, but in a different way. I was a pledge with girls two years younger. Their idea of fun was kidnapping the older members and hiding, giggling all the way.

One of the actives they kidnapped was my old skating partner, Lynne. They took her to a warehouse, tied her to a chair, and put lipstick all over her face. They thought this was hysterically funny. When it was all over, I kept trying to apologize to Lynne, as I had inadvertently led them to her, but she was being whisked off in another car. I told my pledge friends to drop me at my house. Once inside my own home, I burst into tears. Irene came over and watched me. "What happened?" she asked.

"I don't like sororities," I told her. That seemed to be the easiest way to explain.

She went to her room and brought a doll out for me to talk to, in case that might help. I tried to hand the doll back, but Irene said, "You have her sleep with you tonight."

I actually preferred the doll to the pledges.

The next day I called two of my friends in my sorority and told them that I was going to resign. I just didn't fit into their idea of fun. They came to my house right away. "Listen, Terrell, that was just one little isolated thing. Get over it! It's all part of the system. It's how people bond as friends!"

"Are you kidding me? Rush itself was the cruelest thing I've ever seen in my life! Sure, I got invitations in *my* envelope every day. I've lived here forever and people know me. But the girls who came from out of town would find their envelopes empty. They would just stand there, humiliated, tears running down their cheeks. I have never felt so embarrassed or sorry for anyone. It's barbaric, you guys. It's an exclusionary, stupid system. I want no part of it."

One of them said, "You can't stand for anyone to get left out of things, do you realize that?"

"That's right. I can't. Why do you allow it?"

"You're nuts on this subject, do you know that? Life is full of exclusions. Private clubs. Private parties. Not everyone gets included in everything! When are you going to get over that fact?"

I looked up, and Irene was standing in the doorway. I don't know if I had connected the dots yet.

Just then the doorbell rang. It was Lynne. I pulled her inside and put my arms around her. "Will you ever forgive me? What an idiotic mess I got us into. I had no idea—"

"Forgive? Forgive? What's to forgive?" Lynne came into the living room and sat down with the rest of us, laughing. "What an amazing night."

"What are you talking about, Lynne?"

"This is the first time anyone's ever kidnapped me, or actually, the first time anyone's ever even *noticed* me in the sorority. I've been like a transparent ghost for two years! And now we're all friends, even the younger ones!" Lynne had always been about twenty IQ points above us all, and had felt separated out from normal, silly-girl socials. Now she was *in*! She was as happy as I'd ever seen her. I realized I was definitely in the wrong place.

I was still typing my resignation when the phone rang.

Over the crackling, scratchy connection, I could hear Paul, calling from Manila, in the Philippines.

"Hey," he said, "I've got a shore billet. That means I live right here in Manila for two years. We could travel all over the Far East. How about marrying me right away?"

"How soon can you get here?" I asked, opening the drawer and getting out his engagement ring.

Paul came home in early January to pick up three things: two air conditioners and me. We were to be married in our living room on January 5, 1960. At the beginning of the wedding, just before I was to walk down the stairs, Gaylie Anne, one of my nine (!) bridesmaids, lost her contact lens. The wedding march was playing and she was on her hands and knees searching. We all got down on our hands and knees, trying to move the show along and find the lens. Irene got down with us, asking, "What we doing?"

"We're looking for Gaylie Anne's lens," I told her. "It fell out of her eye."

Irene cocked her head. She looked hard at Gaylie Anne. "Her eye is still there."

"No, no honey. Her eye didn't fall out. Just the . . . oh, never mind." The wedding march played on. The father of the bride came up the stairs, saying, "Did you change your mind, Terrell? It's okay if you did."

We explained our problem. Dad went downstairs, and finally Gaylie Anne gave up and we all marched down, Gaylie Anne sort of feeling her way along the wall.

Irene loved being a bridesmaid and loved Paul. She wanted to catch my bouquet and stood at the ready. But she was upstaged by Jeannie's father, who told the group he was tired of supporting her, and presented her with a pair of Keds so she could run fast and beat everyone out for the bouquet. Everyone was laughing. When I went to throw it, he kept yelling, "Come on, Jeannie! You can do it! Catch the bouquet, Jeannie!" Jeannie grabbed it. Her father cheered. Then, laughing, Jeannie gave the bouquet to Irene.

Paul and I spent our first night at the Hotel Utah before taking off for San Francisco and the Philippines. When he carried me across the threshold of our hotel room, I gasped. "You've got to be kidding!"

"What? What's wrong?" he asked.

"Paul, look! We're in the Gene Autry Suite!" And on the table in the living room was a big basket of fruit, all wrapped in cellophane and tied with a red bow. I had made the big time.

Our two years in the Philippines, where Paul worked in the Military Sea Transportation Service, felt like a long honeymoon. I wrote for *Free World* magazine, sponsored by the U.S. Information Service. I taught English to diplomats from the Cuban and Argentinean embassies. We traveled to Hong Kong and Japan. We made lifelong friends in the navy. And at the end of our tour of duty, we came home through Thailand, India, Israel, Egypt, and Europe.

Just before Christmas, we arrived home in Salt Lake. Irene threw her arms around us and said, "Hello, my brother!" to Paul as she hugged him.

We found a little cottage in the Cottonwood area, and I became pregnant with my first baby, Katy, who was born the following Halloween.

Everyone in the family hovered around the baby, including Irene, who held her expertly, since she normally cradled a doll most days of her life.

When Katy was just three months old, the company Paul worked for opened a branch office in Denver and Paul was transferred there. I was sad to leave, and my family was sad to see their first grandchild go, but it was not forever.

Mom and Dad decided to build a new home, smaller, on one level. There would be a room for Bam and one for Irene. They found a lot high above the State Capitol Building, with a dazzling view of Salt Lake Valley. Mother got busy with her fabrics and floor plans, and Dad, who was thinking of retiring, looked forward to a new, quiet life working in his garden with his raspberries and tomatoes and taking some classes at the university. He would find somewhere for Irene to live as she got old enough to leave home. And all would be well.

I just love how we cling to hope and illusion.

6

Tilting at Windmills

Parents of disabled children tackle little problems every hour—problems other parents just don't have in their lives. But the biggie, the nagging worry that looms foremost in their subconscious, is, of course, how will my child cope when I'm gone?

For Dad, this came more and more into his conscious mind as he saw Bam aging, Mother's arthritis worsening, and his own energy flagging.

One evening, while Paul and I were still living in Denver, Dad sat down and announced a plan to Mom and Bammy.

"I want us to take a trip to California, to a place called the Devereux School. It's near Santa Barbara and overlooks the sea. It's a residential school for young people like Irene. It looks very nice. Rosemary Kennedy, Jack Kennedy's sister, lives at the one on the East Coast."

"Send her away?" Mom asked plaintively. "It would be like sending a three-year-old away."

"We spoil her, all of us. Bammy waits on her hand and foot. If she knocks a vase over, Bammy cleans it up. She constantly interrupts people to get attention, and you force everyone to pay attention to her, and it ruins any hope of table conversation. Honey, we are crippling her chances of surviving in the world."

"She won't know what to do without us!"

"That's right. And she'll have to learn. That's the whole point. It doesn't have to be forever. Just until she learns some independence. We aren't always going to be around to baby her. Devereux is expensive. I can afford it for at least five years, and maybe that's all she'll need. Or maybe she'll love it there so much by then that she'll want to stay, and then I'll have to figure out if I can afford that."

And so it was that Irene, at age twenty, went to the Devereux School near Santa Barbara, California. Despite the lovely campus by the sea, Mom was in mourning and worried. Bam was relieved, and Dad was relishing the freedom. All would be well at last. If only he could make enough money to care for Irene at Devereux for the rest of her life, this burden would be lifted from his—and our—shoulders.

Of course, if you want to make God laugh, the saying goes, tell him your plans.

NATURALLY, IRENE DID NOT want to stay at Devereux. She had a roommate, which really disturbed her. "Mom, I like my privacy," she said. None of us even knew that she knew the word "privacy." But Dad was firm: Irene must learn more independence. A few years down the road, maybe she could have a place of her own back in her own hometown, but for now, this would be good for her. The Devereux staff seemed professional, compassionate, and very dedicated to these young people. The campus was lovely and there were walking trails to the beach. The living quarters were clean and spacious. The program included talent shows, arts and crafts, dances and parties, and outings into Santa Barbara. You couldn't ask for more. But of course it had been a terrible wrench saying good-bye to Irene and driving away as she waved good-bye, crying, from the front porch of her dorm, even though a staff member at Devereux had her arm around her.

Shortly after leaving Irene, Mom and Dad flew to Denver to be near us and get some solace. They reported all the events at Devereux. Paul and I told them they certainly deserved some time to themselves, and Irene really needed independence from this overindulgent family. We loved her, we protected her, we spoiled her. She was twenty. It was high time.

We had news for them, too: I was pregnant again. They were delighted, but so longing to be in the same city with their grandchildren.

Our second daughter was born in Denver six months later, four days before Christmas. We had to spend Christmas Day in the hospital because the baby's big sister, Katy, two years older, had a horrible ear infection that week, and the pediatrician said we needed to give the baby a fighting chance at home and let Katy get over her ear infection. Bammy called Paul from Salt Lake. "I'm flying over right away. Meet me at the airport. We'll tell Katy Christmas is two days later. She'll never know the difference. I'm not going to have my baby Katy neglected while you take care of the little one." Paul picked Bammy up and Katy flew into the arms of her great-grandmother, who immediately cuddled her and started telling her stories. That night, Paul heard the creak of the rocking chair and Bammy's voice once again singing "Red River Valley."

They treated Christmas like any other day, and Bammy told Kate that Santa would be coming soon. Two days after Christmas, I brought home our new daughter, Marriott, which is Paul's middle name. (His mother was sister to Bill and seven other Marriotts, but unfortunately we did not own any hotel stock!)

We made December 27 Christmas then, and Bammy fixed her wonderful Danish *ableskivers* for breakfast, running with butter and her homemade raspberry jam.

Back in Salt Lake, Irene was home for Christmas vacation with Mom and Dad. She got off the plane in her pretty traveling suit, looking pulled-together and radiantly happy, Mom told me on the phone. They had a fine visit together, and then it was time for Irene to get on the plane. Apparently her radiant happiness was because she was home. Returning to Devereux was another matter.

"No! I don't like it there! I don't want to go back," Irene wailed. Mom started to cry. Dad was firm. "Yes, but you are going back, Irene. Remember how Terrell went to Stanford and had a bedroom there, and roommates and everything? This is *your* turn now."

Dad, like all of us, continued to labor under the illusion that you can reason with Irene.

How they got her in the car and onto the plane, I'll never know. I'm just thrilled I was nursing a new baby in Denver and Bammy was tending her big sister, far removed from Irene's piteous cries not to be sent away again.

During our three years in Denver, Paul was away on business

for weeks at a time and I learned how to be a single mom. Again we made lifelong friends, this time with our neighbors, who took me under their wing in all sorts of ways. We had a German shepherd, who drove me so crazy I wrote a humor piece about him, just to get my frustration out. It was a habit I began to adopt when things went wrong in the house, or with the kids or with the car. If it drove us nuts, I found the humor in it and wrote it down. I kept a little file of pieces written when things were so bad there was nothing to do but laugh about it. Paul and I have shared that habit over the years. When we are at our wit's end, one of us starts to shake with laughter.

Then, in 1966, Paul was called back to Salt Lake to work in the home office of the company. Mom and Dad were overjoyed. We found a lovely home on Third Avenue, one block from Paul's childhood home.

When they told me who had owned the house at one time, I nearly fainted. It was the doctor who had delivered Irene, the one that Bammy had cursed so often for not being more helpful to Mom. "What ever happened to him?" I asked the realtor.

"Oh, it's so sad. He is down at the state mental hospital. Been there for years. Just went insane and never got well." I could hardly wait to tell Bammy. She would nod her head and quietly discuss divine justice.

I also wrote a piece about the horrors of moving and finally sent it, along with my piece about the dog, to one of our local papers, just to see if anyone was interested. To my surprise and joy, the features editor called back and said they wanted them. I asked how she felt about my doing one a week for them. She quickly responded: "Yes! Let's do it! What would you like to call your column?"

I wanted to be free to write about anything, and so I stole a title of one Robert Benchley's books, silently asking his late spirit to forgive me. I said, "Let's call it *Of All Things.*" My first column appeared in the *Desert News* on June 7, 1967. Just as my column appeared in print, Dorothy Parker, Robert Benchley's partner and girlfriend, died. I have no idea what any of it means, karmicly.

The column ran on Mondays for thirteen years, and in all that time, I didn't mention Irene. I couldn't get the right tone with her as a subject. The last thing I wanted to do was make fun of her, although I regularly made fun of my husband and children as well as myself. In fact, my family was hurt when they and their latest activities didn't appear in the column.

When my first byline appeared in the paper, the folks in the Association for Retarded Children—ARC—remembered me from our family's earlier work. They called me right up to ask my help in promoting still more programs for the mentally disabled. "We know Irene's in California, but you never know when you might want her to come home again and be part of her home-town community," they said. Knowing my parents' commitment to this project, they just assumed I would pitch in and help. I felt as if I'd just had an offer I couldn't refuse.

From the time we swept out the first day care center when I was twelve, I knew these families, and now their children were grown up and had nowhere to go during the day. Their parents were aging and worried. They certainly didn't want to send these grown children to live in the state institution after all these years in the community.

What we needed was a sheltered workshop for adults, such as the Flame of Hope workshops that the Kennedys had founded a few years before. We organized ourselves and researched the Salt Lake community for buildings no one wanted anymore. We found an elementary school that was being closed, and asked the school district if we could use it if we maintained it, and they agreed. For money for maintenance and staff, we asked foundations, individuals, the Junior League. We had a plan in mind: start the program, then get the school district to take it over. Why would they do that? Because in our plan we had in mind passing a law that guaranteed free public education to *all* Utah's children, mentally disabled or not. But we kept that part quiet for now. First things first.

We opened Columbus Community Center, a sheltered workshop for teens and adults with mental disabilities, on June 6, 1968. As I drove to the center, I learned that Bobby Kennedy had died from the gunshot wound he had received the day before. Wiping my tears and blowing my nose, I arrived at the room where our first clients sat around a table, working on a craft. Two were in wheelchairs. I looked carefully at all of them, trying to see their leader. "Hello, guys!" I said to them in a high, patronizing voice you use for little children. "Are you having fun here?"

They looked up at me blankly.

"Where is your, um, supervisor?" I asked a very large young woman in a wheelchair.

"You're looking at her," she answered levelly.

She should have thrown something at me for being so stupid, but she just smiled and held out her hand and introduced herself. I apologized to her, and she waved it off. Then she introduced me to the first clients. They each shook my hand and smiled. This was a good sign. They were busy, they had someplace to go every day, and they would make new friends.

The man we had hired to run Columbus Community Center was Glenn Latham, who went on to become one of the best behavior modification specialists in the country. One of the first clients, Jerry Deming, was a thirty-five-year-old man who did not speak and was so hyperactive he tried to climb walls and curtains. Glenn found out from Jerry's mom what Jerry loved most, which was Junior Mints. His mother took him into Glenn's office, and Glenn watched him bouncing off walls. Glenn caught Jerry sitting still for one second and popped a Junior Mint in his mouth. Jerry jumped up, jubilant, and ran around the room again. Glenn waited. The moment Jerry got tired and sat down for a second, another mint was put into his mouth. This made Jerry experiment a little. He ran around the room once and sat down. He got a mint. He jumped from his chair and sat down again, fast, and got two mints. Chewing thoughtfully, he simply looked at Glenn and waited. Three more mints.

By the end of the day, Jerry had stopped running and climbing. That afternoon, when Mrs. Deming came to Glenn's office to see which padded cell he'd had to leave Jerry in, she found Jerry sitting quietly in Glenn's office, his legs crossed, reading a magazine. The magazine was upside down, but Jerry was totally quiet and calm.

It took Glenn Latham twelve minutes to change Jerry's life. And no, Jerry didn't overdose on Junior Mints. The intervals between bad behaviors became longer and longer, and eventually he switched to tokens, which could be exchanged for goodies from the Columbus "store." Glenn went on to do the same thing with hundreds of others like Jerry.

What we learned from Glenn Latham was this: Catch people

doing something right, reward them, and you will have them in the palm of your hand.

I brought that little trick home with me. When Paul helped me clear the table, I said, "Thank you so much, honey. That really helps." He did it more often.

My daughter Marriott was four at the time and wanted to be go ice skating with me. I really love to skate, but my idea of skating is flying along to good music. Marriott's idea was that I would hold her up under both arms so she would feel safe, thereby almost breaking my back.

Thanks to my behavior modification training, I went to the snack bar and bought a small bag of M&M's. I took Mare out on the ice and told her to just stand there. Frowning and fussing, she did. We just stood there for a minute, then one of Marriott's feet moved just slightly forward. "Hey! Did you see that? Look what you did! How did you *do* that?" I said, popping an M&M into her mouth. She thought for a moment. Then her other foot moved maybe three inches. Another M&M went in her mouth. "Yes! Yes!"

I waited. She looked at me. Then she tentatively, purposefully, moved her first foot forward, got a reward, and then brought the other foot along, and was again rewarded, all the while getting lavish praise from me.

She was doing a little skating shuffle all around the rink by herself, and I was able to skate with a pain-free back.

Within six months, Marriott could do little twizzles on the ice, and she was always the best skater at her friends' skating parties. Her teeth were rotting, but, boy, could she skate!

Meanwhile, it was time to start our next phase of the plan: let mentally disabled children go to school with normal children.

At first the whole idea sent the parents of normal children, and their teachers, into a state of panic. How could a teacher accommodate this in a classroom? The answer came from stacks of research, much of it in Europe, pointing out that the mentally disabled make up about 3 percent of any population; so if you have a classroom of thirty "normal" children, chances are you'll have only one mentally disabled one. If you as a teacher do nothing but just let him sit there, he will absorb the behaviors of the other children and start to improve and learn little bits on his own. Contrast that idea with bundling all special-needs kids into the same room, where they each pick up the others' odd behaviors and learn more odd behavior.

It was an idea whose time had come. Pennsylvania had already passed a law allowing this to become a reality. We wanted Utah to be next.

How could we convince everyone to let all children go to school? We decided to apply Glenn Latham's behavior modification treatment to government officials, reporters, and legislators: we caught them doing something right and thanked the hell out of them. If a reporter put something good about our programs on the news that night, we would instigate a phone-calling or letter-writing campaign to thank him for his incredibly insightful report. If a legislator spoke even one sentence of approval for our ideas, she would get notes and calls of praise.

This startled the legislators and heads of government, who were used to receiving only criticism and pleading. Pretty soon, whenever they'd see us in the halls of the legislature, or in their waiting rooms, or in the newspaper offices, they'd say, "Well, hi. What can I do for you?"

With that sort of support, we were able to convince the Utah

Legislature to pass House Bill 105 in January 1969, entitling *all* children to a free public education, including the mentally disabled.

After a few years' hard work on the part of parents in all over the country in the ARC, Congress passed Public Law 94–142 in 1975, and now every state had to follow suit.

We in Utah even went so far as to suggest that special-needs children who lived far from school needed to be taken by bus, the way the other children were. The school district officials agreed, after much praise from us all for their caring foresight.

The head of the bus company at the time, Charles Boynton, was nervous about being able to get enough buses and competent drivers to handle all these kids. But at the end of the first day of service, Charlie called me and said, "Well, we did it. We only have three sack lunches, two apples, and one kid left over." (The kid was rescued shortly, happy as could be that he got to ride on a real bus by himself.)

We didn't stop at just sending Charlie a thank-you note. We decided on a grander idea, a better way to thank all the people who cared for this cause as much as we did.

We decided to hold an awards luncheon every year. We would call it the Don Quixote Luncheon, because many people felt that pushing for community programs for people whose brains were damaged was definitely just tilting at windmills.

Fifty people showed up at the luncheon. I welcomed them, and after lunch I introduced Robert Peterson, a magnificent and well-loved baritone actor who had appeared as Lancelot on Broadway and starred in *Man of La Mancha* locally many times. He thanked everyone in the room for what they did for mentally disabled citizens. When he sang "The Impossible

Dream," a lot of hankies came out. Then we awarded our little wooden statues of Don Quixote to a variety of people who had done major things for us that year: a legislator, a TV reporter, a small-business owner who hired a special-needs person part-time, and, of course, Charlie the bus man. We described all the good they had done. We clapped for them. I still see our little wooden statues in offices downtown.

Another thing we did in those years was make close friends with the local and state officials who ran services for groups that might include the mentally retarded. We invited them to speak at our local and regional conventions. One year, at a meeting in a mountain resort in Colorado, we made good friends with Evan Jones, a very intelligent, friendly man who ran the Division of Family Services for Utah. Over dinner one night, he announced that he didn't think he could support our programs completely the following year, owing to budget restrictions.

We told him, laughing, that there would be consequences if he did not include every soul who needed services. He said supporting all the programs we wanted was going to be impossible.

That night, some of our group entered his hotel room and short-sheeted his bed. How they got into his room, I'll never know. I was horrified. But the next day at the luncheon, where he was the speaker, he spoke of the hazards of working with folks in the ARC, who were bent on doing right by our citizens who could not speak for themselves. He then reported the short-sheeting and laughed. It was very curious: for some reason, instead of being insulted and offended, he felt pleased to be a part of our riotous little gang.

And oh yes, P.S.: we got most of the people on the list served that year. We learned there are many ways to get things done.

Nationally, parents in other states were matching our work stride for stride (though possibly they drew the line at short-sheeting beds). It was exciting work and we considered our job done. These young people and adults would be cared for in day programs always and forever.

We were so naïve. We didn't realize it takes eternal vigilance.

7

The Spies Who Loved Community

"Never doubt," said Margaret Mead, "that a small group of thoughtful, committed citizens can change the world. Indeed, it is the only thing that ever has." She also said that in those years the National Association for Retarded Citizens was the most effective voluntary action group in the country. I was honored to be invited to be on their national board, and I traveled to meetings twice a year and enjoyed every second of it.

Mom worried that I was spending too much time on this effort when I could be doing other things. "What other things?" I asked.

"Well, you're a writer."

"I'm writing a column a week! What more could you want?"

"Well, I don't want you to neglect your children or husband."

"Mom, we're fine. I'm the Brownie leader! My girls are not neglected."

"Your own daughter just resigned from the Brownie troop."

"Now don't pin that on *me*. Marriott is not a joiner. I can't help that."

Dad worried too. "Irene's away at Devereux now. Why would you put so much effort into this movement when you don't have to?"

"Dad, listen to me. I did not finish my Stanford education, and I'm still doing dribs and drabs of classes to graduate from the University of Utah sometime in this century. I want you to know that I am now getting the education of my life, on how politics work, how you get bills through the legislature, how you effect social change. Stanford was *nothing* compared to this."

It was true. I learned more about how government works by being a volunteer with this group than I ever could by taking political science in college. This was front-line stuff. I learned who the players were and how to make friends and influence people. I reminded Dad of Bobby Kennedy's famous campaign question, which he applied to the whole nation as he ran for president: "If not us, who? If not now, when?" That's how this work felt for me and for the folks I worked with.

Irene was still at Devereux. Mom and Dad and I went to visit her one family weekend when she was in the chorus of *The Mikado.* She proudly showed us around backstage, and then took us to her room, which she shared with another girl. I could see the girl hurry to leave as Irene came in. The room was neat and clean. We had hopes, for just a minute, that Irene was happy there. But then she sat down on the bed and said, "When I'm coming home to live with you again?"

"Honey, don't you like it here?" Mom asked, sitting down by her and putting an arm around her.

"I want my own room, Mom."

Our hearts hurt. We all want a room of our own.

Later, when we met with her staff, we learned that she hit her roommate often. They had tried bribery, withholding of privileges, everything they could think of to stop the behavior, but it wasn't working. Also, they had to shower her every morning, instead of letting her take her own showers. They said her personal hygiene was just not good, that she needed to wash the parts of the body that needed it, and she never did. She screamed every time they did it for her.

I think I would, too. But how else could she keep clean?

We left her there, but I knew Irene would love to have the chance to live in her own community and not be isolated on a campus far away, pretty as it was. Mentally disabled adults whose parents are aging and dying need community group homes.

In Utah in those years, most of the state funding for the mentally disabled was sent to the state training school in Utah County. A certain state senator from that county had most of his family members working at the school. The idea of allowing the communities to set up group homes for this population would be okay, *as long as it was funneled through the state institution*. One always wants first cut of the money, of course.

So the state institution had a complete hammerlock on all community services, and the officials dragged their feet on setting up any services outside Utah County. The good senator even thought of a hugely expensive park and playground "for all of Utah's handicapped children." It would, of course, be placed *on the grounds of the state institution!* And even more marvelous was that the man chosen to head up this grand new park was the senator's brother.

It seemed a perfect idea to the senator, who was very power-ful in the legislature and had a lot of favors to call in. While our group tried our best to explain that physically and mentally handicapped children would really like to play in their local parks like everyone else, our voices were summarily dismissed and the park funding sailed on through. Our dream of group homes in communities all over the state was fading fast.

But we were wrong. The National Association for Retarded Citizens, bless their fantastic little hearts, working in Washing-ton with Congress, sent something our way that changed every-thing forever.

It was a grant application. It was called Projects of National Significance: Community Alternatives to Institutionalization. Only community people could apply. Not institution people. It came to our Council for Developmental Disabilities, whose ex-ecutive director, Elizabeth Lowe, saw the whole picture of insti-tution versus community clearly and saw her chance to help us.

We had nothing going for us except a passion for community programs and the help of Elizabeth, along with one other spy inside state government, Geri Clark, who had orchestrated all the arrangements for Columbus Community Center from behind the scenes in the state board of education. Geri had also master-minded the passing of the bill that allowed the mentally disabled to attend school.

Late one night, Geri Clark got a phone call from Elizabeth Lowe. She was whispering, as if the senator and his family might be tapping her phone. And she told Geri about the grant. "Who can write this fast and get it in the mail by midnight Monday? And it has to be signed by the governor."

I was home saying good night to the girls. Geri called me and said, "Elizabeth will meet you at the Hotel Utah coffee shop at eight a.m. and hand you a grant application. Grab it and get out to my house immediately."

"Oh, okay," said I. We had all learned to take orders from Geri. She was just like the Godfather. "What's it for, and are you going to write it?"

"It's for group homes, run by the community, and no, you are going to write it."

"I have never written a grant in my life."

"There's a first time for everything. See you about eight-thirty."

Geri had been so good, so successful at getting done what needed to be done, you just didn't say no to her. I canceled all my plans for the next day and in the morning met Elizabeth, who quickly handed me the application as if handing over a spy document, and hurried away.

Geri and I waded through the instructions. The grant seemed as long as a Tolstoy novel to us. We had absolutely no idea what we were doing. She kept pouring coffee for me, fixing me soup and toast, and telling me, "You can do this." We used the model of the Eastern Nebraska Community of Retardation, ENCOR, which had started the whole ball rolling three years before, using the research of a French outfit called L'ARCH. The French showed the amazing progress and financial savings that happen when you give mentally disabled people a chance to live in their own communities in the least restrictive environment. These group homes were staffed by young French people who loved being able to make a difference in the world. It was a model that changed the world for mentally disabled people. The key phrase was "least restrictive environment." Well, don't we all want that?

We wrote and wrote for a week. My children went to school looking ragged. Paul did what laundry he could, and burgers and pizza were our fare. Every day for a week, I drove out to Geri's and she fed me and urged me on. At night I would take it home and rewrite, trying to fit in all the buzzwords they wanted: independence, new skills for community living, integration into community, and so on. I must have managed three hours of sleep a night, but by Sunday night I retyped the whole thing (this was long before computers), and on Monday I called Dad.

I told him what I had been writing. I told him it was vital for all the kids like Irene, and I needed him to call Governor Cal Rampton, who knew and liked Dad, and tell him we needed his signature by tonight. Remembering how our group had hounded the governor with all our letters urging change, I wasn't sure he'd see me alone.

Dad listened, hearing the exhaustion in my voice, and said, "Okay. I'll call you right back." He and Cal Rampton had known each other a long time.

That evening we went up to the State Capitol Building, where the governor was working late. Dad took his watch off and put it on the governor's desk. "Cal, I am going to take exactly seven minutes of your time, and then leave you be. You know I don't ask you for many favors, but I'm asking one tonight. Listen to my daughter."

I explained what we had in front of us. I told the governor that by starting this project, we would be starting a new phase in caring for the disabled, in their own communities.

"This system of group homes will cost about half of what institutionalization costs," I told him. (Current costs for institutions per person: $410 per day; community group homes: $250 per day, in Utah, anyway.)

"If you get it, it will probably break the back of the institution," he said.

"That's right, Governor. In time that will probably happen." My heart pounded. I knew the parents' groups had annoyed him with so many letters.

The governor rolled his office chair around to stare out at the valley for a minute. Then he slowly turned it back, looking through his bushy eyebrows at Dad and me. "And you know this is going to infuriate a certain senator, don't you?"

"Yes, sir," I said.

Smiling, he took out his pen.

"Let's do it and see what happens," he said.

"Thank you, Governor," Dad said, taking his watch back. We shook hands and Dad drove me to the post office, where we mailed it before the midnight deadline.

At the next meeting of the Developmental Disabilities Council, a delighted Elizabeth Lowe announced that the Utah ARC had been awarded an $85,000 grant for community group homes. The head of the state institution turned four shades of purple, stood, and slapped the table. "Why was I not informed about this grant?"

"Look at the title of the grant," I told him, and handed it to him. "It's "Community Alternatives to Institutionalization." Community people had to apply."

A lot of murmuring, shouting, and head shaking went on as

the institution people had a little tantrum. Then we ended the meeting. Community group homes would become a reality.

We called ourselves Project TURN: Teaching Utah's Retarded Normalization. The parent who named Project TURN, Fran Peek, was the father of Kim, who was attending Columbus Community Center. Kim can remember everything he's ever read, and his mind counts like an adding machine. He is a walking encyclopedia of facts, dates, and names that he never forgets. His favorite reading at that time was phone books from any city, which he'd read in a couple of hours and memorize completely. The staff at Columbus saw the possibilities in Kim, and he became their filer and office payroll chief. He could do all these things, but in between, would hum and look hard at the palm of his hand. With all his talents, Kim could not dress or bathe himself.

In the future, Kim would go on to make history.

Kim's condition is now called "prestigious intellectual megamemory savant." Fran and Kim were attending a national ARC meeting and met screenwriter Barry Morrow who had heard some of the amazing stories about Kim's mind. "I want to make a movie about this," Barry told Kim's father.

Soon Kim found Dustin Hoffman following him around for weeks, learning Kim's behaviors for the role of Raymond Babbit. *Rain Man* won five academy awards. At the premiere, Kim said, "Hi, Dustin. You're the star!" Dustin wrapped his arms around Kim and said, "I may be the star, Kim, but you are the heavens." Dustin told Fran, "You've got to share this guy with the world." And Fran has done just that: working with special-education teachers, they developed a plan to teach students and everyone that "it's okay to be different, because everybody is different."

Kim and Fran have interacted with over 4 million people world-wide in the past nineteen years, and have logged nearly 2 million miles. Kim lets everyone hold Dustin's Oscar, which Dustin gave to Kim.

But in the late 1970s, people were still afraid of people who were "different." For us working on Project TURN, convincing the neighbors that we would be good neighbors, too, was an experience in itself. We have battle scars from neighborhood meetings. "Not in My Back Yard!" became the worn slogan heard over and over. Trying to convince people that retarded people are okay was a challenge. ("But just because he looked funny walking down the sidewalk, Mrs. Parsons, didn't mean he was drunk and disorderly, really. That's just the way he walks. You didn't need to call the police. He was just going to his bus stop to go to work.")

The police learned to know and protect these citizens and became their true friends. Slowly the neighbors came around to realizing these were not criminals living next door. Soon the project rented groups of apartments where these citizens could live with minimal supervision.

Things were falling into place for many of the nation's mentally disabled. And Irene was still safely tucked away at Devereux in California. I could finally relax and follow some other interests, including my girls, my writing, and my husband. Mom, Dad, and Bammy were still free of the nagging day-to-day worry of Irene's care. I could finally concentrate on my family and my writing. We were all going to live happily ever after.

And God was doubled over, laughing, calling her friends to hear this one.

8

Eviction Is Such an Ugly Word

Dear Mr. and Mrs. Harris:

We are sorry to report that we must send Irene home from Devereux. Our staff has done all it can to prevent her tantrums and hitting her roommate, but we have finally come to the conclusion that it is in the best interests of our other clients to terminate Irene's stay with us. We have done our very best over these six years, but we see now that perhaps others in your community may be better equipped to handle her. We have tried medications, but they have not been effective in controlling her outbursts. We will terminate her stay with us one month from now, and hope you will be able to make further arrangements on your end.

Sincerely,

The Devereux School Staff
Goleta, California

I've had to paraphrase here, because we lost that letter a long time ago. But that was the gist of it. The Devereux schools are a godsend to many families. They have fine facilities and caring staff. I have wished many times that Irene had been happy there. My life would have been very different if she had.

A month later, when Mom and Dad picked up Irene and all her suitcases to drive her home, she was beaming with delight. Back at home, Bammy was wringing her hands and wondering how much strength she had left to care for Irene daily.

But, *TA-DA!* Good news, Bammy—we now have a group home program! Thanks to short-sheeting Evan Jones's bed, and possibly other enticements such as funding from the legislature, his Office of Family Services contracted with Project TURN to provide group-home placements. Irene was eligible to enter that program, I told Bam. I know we can find a place for Irene there. I worked hard on that project! They'll surely make a place for her.

And they did.

And it lasted three whole months.

Irene wanted to come home, and she knew exactly how to get there.

She threw a couch through a plateglass window. Well, it was a love seat, and she didn't actually throw it: she pushed it so hard that it broke the window.

The staff, being well trained in behavior modification, ignored it.

It's really hard to ignore a couch slamming through a plateglass window.

But they turned their backs on her, because you're supposed to ignore inappropriate behavior and reward appropriate behavior. Turning your back on a broken bay window with a couch sticking through it demonstrated their earnest attempts at coping with Irene.

Noticing that she hadn't received their complete attention, Irene then sat down on the floor and took off her shoes and socks and bit her big toe so hard that blood spurted out.

This they could not ignore.

They called me up and explained sorrowfully they had failed with her, and for the sake of the other residents, they had to expel her.

Irene had won again. She was back on my parents' doorstep, absolutely thrilled. For Irene, the best news of all, besides moving home again, was that Mom and Dad had built a small swimming pool, so that Mom could walk in it to ease her arthritic joints. When they finally filled the brand-new pool with water on the first warm day in spring, Irene climbed into her bathing suit.

My two daughters were there with Mom, and all three of them said, "Irene, you can't get in yet! We have to wait two more days until it gets heated up enough!"

"I want to go in now! Now!" she pleaded, heading for the pool.

"Irene," Mom said, "honey, it's freezing. You have to wait."

"No! No! It's not cold for me!" Irene started hitting herself, biting her knuckle, her whole routine.

Mom had simply had it. "Okay, sweetie. Fine. See for yourself."

Irene ran to the pool and jumped in. When her head came up, she was gasping for breath. The girls ran to get a towel, and Irene climbed right out. As they tried to warm and console her, she snapped, "Don't breathe on me!"

Now when my girls are freezing cold, they say to each other, "Don't breathe on me!"

Mother loved being able to watch over Irene again, Dad was making triple manhattans, and Bammy? Well, Bammy had her own ways of living life.

Bammy survived by caring for all of us and playing bridge with her friends. Her morning routine consisted of serving Mom breakfast in bed and then pulling on Dad's galoshes for garden work, this all still in her nightgown. Every summer morning we would see Bam out in the garden, weeding, in her nightgown and Dad's galoshes. In winter, she pulled on the galoshes so that she could go out and wash the family car in the garage. Our washer and dryer were out in the garage, too. She could clean house, weed the garden, wash the car, and then put a load of laundry in before she ran down the hall to her bath to get ready for her bridge lunch. Knowing Dad was at work, she would often just pop her nightgown in the wash and run naked down the hall to the bathroom.

One icy winter day, Mom was driving Irene to her workshop. In the garage, Bam put her nightgown in the wash, which was already in progress. Then, naked except for Dad's galoshes, she went to go in the door to the house. Somehow the door had locked itself from the inside. Bam was trapped in the garage. Her nightgown was irretrievable. She had no choice but to push the button to open the garage door, race around to the front door, find the key in the flower pot, and let herself back in. Except that just as she reached the front door, she heard the mailman whistling up the sidewalk, behind the scrub oak branches. She raced around to the side of the house and crouched down, shivering. When he finally left, she padded through the snow to the front door and let herself in, only slightly the worse for the wear.

When Irene came home from Columbus that day, saying she'd had to spend a lot of time in the time-out room for hitting a coworker, Bammy told her, "You don't even know what a bad day is."

But of course Irene did know, and every day of the eighteen years she spent at Columbus Community Center, with dozens of others like her, was hell for her in many ways. Her constant need for individual attention drove her to tantrums and violence against the others. Like many people with developmental disabilities, she wants to be the only one in the room with the problem. So she did spend a lot of time alone in the time-out room. And in those years, the drugs available for this sort of behavior were just not known or available.

It was during this time that Mom appeared one morning at my house. I offered her coffee and kept on doing the breakfast dishes, because I was due at a meeting soon. Mom put her head in her hands and started to sob. I went over to her and put my arms around her. "What is it, Mom?"

"I'm so discouraged, I don't know what to do. Irene doesn't fit in anywhere, and I can't cope with her anymore. I don't want to leave her to you to have to deal with. I'm thinking the best solution is to just kill her somehow, and then kill myself."

I hugged her some more and then went back to my dishes. "Mom, I don't think that's a good solution. Really."

"Well, I don't see any way out." She put her head in her arms on the table and sobbed some more. The more she dramatized her sadness, the more quiet and numb I became.

I wiped the counters and said, "Hang on for a while. Things change. Something will come up. A door will open."

She seemed to want me to join her in her tears, but I couldn't. I think I had developed a core of stoicism over the years, maybe because Mom seemed to cry a lot. Maybe I was always thinking hard how to fix it. But I didn't cry or rage, at least on the outside.

"Mom, I'm really sorry. I have to go to a meeting." She stood up, hugged me, and said she was sorry, too.

As I drove to the meeting, I felt really sad, first for Mom and then for myself. I simply couldn't think of how to help her with her despair.

Mom did not kill herself, or Irene. Irene's days were spent at Columbus Community Center, but she was at home with Mom, Dad, and Bammy every other minute and on weekends, needing constant supervision and expecting constant attention. They were getting too old for this.

During this time, Paul and I would bring our two daughters to Mom, Dad, and Bam's new house high above the Capitol in Salt Lake for dinner. Irene, always delighted to see her nieces, would come out holding one of her dolls. Even at age two and four, my children could see that Irene was not like normal adults. When they asked to see her doll, she would start to hit herself and yell, "No! It's mine!"

It seemed a little odd to them for a grown woman to be acting like this. I remember that one of the first times it happened, I was able to get them alone in another room for a minute. Their sweet, intelligent little faces were looking at me for guidance, ready for an explanation. "When Irene was born, she had something go wrong in her brain. It got hurt, and it can't be fixed. She can't read and write, the way you are going to as you grow up. She needs us to take care of her and help her all we can."

They nodded, accepting my explanation. They sometimes took her hand and led her into their bedrooms to see their own dolls or other toys. She loved seeing their playthings, and never tried to take them. She just couldn't bring herself to share her own toys. But when it was time for a daughter's birthday party, I was always in a bind. Should I include Irene, who loved the parties and the balloons, and our local baker Mrs. Backer's famous birthday cakes? Or could I take a pass and just concentrate on my children and their friends? In those two or three years when Irene was living back at home, I felt I had to invite her, especially since my mom was always an integral part of the parties. My mother loved parties, she helped me with the decorations, and my children adored her. They called her Rosie, and she added to their parties with little touches that made them memorable. Since Katy was born on Halloween, Mom became a masked fortune-teller, reading palms by candlelight. The children delighted in her act and looked forward to it.

But when Irene came, it was a bit of an embarrassment to the little girls. They tried their best, but it's hard, when you're turning four or five or six, to be compassionate and grown-up and introduce your strange aunt to your friends. (I once heard one of them telling a friend, "My aunt has a broken brain. But she is nice, too, and we love her.")

Irene, of course, wanted to open the presents. We stopped her, but then she wanted to fish in the fish pond for the favors. I'd be standing behind the sheet, hooking the tiny gifts on the fishing string, praying that the little person on the other end of the fishing pole was not a really big person who pushed to the front of the line.

Looking back on it, I think it marvelous that my daughters put up with all this over those early years. Wait: they had no choice. They had to accept the fact that, yes, this is our aunt. Get over it.

I think these situations helped make them what they are to-day: competent, contributing citizens of their community with an extra dose of compassion. They have taught their own daughters to treat Irene the same loving way they do.

Meanwhile, back at the homestead, Irene was still attending Columbus during the day, spending a lot of time in the time-out room, and living with Mom, Dad, and Bam. But all of a sudden, everyone but me seemed to fall apart all at once. Bammy developed throat cancer; Dad, a smoker since he was eighteen, was diagnosed with emphysema; and Mom got cancer of the bile duct. Once again they had nowhere to turn for help with (and for) Irene.

With a pounding heart, I offered to create a private program for her. I'd find her a live-in companion and an apartment, and she could still take the bus every day to her sheltered workshop. After all, I had helped put other community programs in place. Why couldn't I do a private one for Irene? By this time my parents were so worn down that they agreed. Dad put some of his savings in a trust for her and made me the trustee. "We didn't mean to put this on your shoulders," Dad said.

"God knows I didn't mean to put it on my shoulders either," I told him. "But when you think about it, Dad, we've been training me for this all my life." At least I knew the system and had friends in high and low places who could give me advice.

I felt so noble, standing there, looking at him across the room. He was wearing his oxygen tube and looking at me, his face solemn and concerned. I thought it was because he was in awe of my sacrifice, to help with the Irene situation.

Then he pointed to my feet.

I was standing on his oxygen tube.

I jumped off, and Dad sort of crumbled to a chair and appeared to faint. I ran to him, but he opened his eyes and laughed. "Want to hear the best thing that happened this morning?" he said, sitting up.

"I got a phone call. The fellow said, 'We are raising money to help the disabled.' And I said, 'Oh, thank heavens you've called. I need about five thousand dollars as soon as you can send it.' There was this long pause, and then he hung up." He slapped the couch, laughing.

We advertised in the classifieds for a companion for Irene, and started looking for an apartment for her. Dad, the pro of all pros, wrote the ad. We sought a companion for a mildly retarded young lady who was physically independent. He did not mention that she threw couches through plateglass windows or that her screams could shatter glass. After all, this could be a little surprise to be discovered later, right?

We rented a nice two-bedroom apartment in a complex close to the bus line, and then we waited and prayed. And out of many applicants we found a young woman who was a psychology major at the university. Debbie handled Irene beautifully, and we knew we were home free.

One of our friends who was a lawyer, and who knew Irene well, helped me draw up a contract for Debbie. "Now, how much will you be paying her?" he asked.

"Five hundred," I said.

"Five hundred?" he asked. He'd spent time with Irene at our house. He was not one of the most patient people in the world. "Yes, but how often?" He suggested that five hundred daily or even hourly might get the job done, if we were lucky.

While we made plans for Irene's future, the Fourth of July

came around, and we thought Irene should come with us to the church picnic just up the hill from our house. Children rolled on the grassy slope, fried chicken and hot dogs sizzled on the grill, a long table of great potato salads and ten different flavors of home-made ice cream beckoned. In the corner of the lawn stood a little stage where the bishop could give a talk, praising the birth of our country and all it stands for. Paul and I got busy talking with old friends. The children began to play with their new friends. Teenagers had been assigned to look out for the little ones, so Marriott even had a supervisor with a puppet on her hand.

The only person without something to do or someone to talk to was Irene. This did not faze her for a moment.

The next thing I heard was the crowd being told to be quiet. Maybe the bishop was going to speak. I turned to see Irene stand-ing on the stage with the bishop, who was announcing that it was Irene Harris's birthday, and now everyone joined in to sing to her. She was simply beaming.

When she climbed down from the stage amidst all the friendly and loving applause, I finally reached her. "Irene, look at me. When is your birthday?"

"March twenty-fourth," she replied.

"Is this March twenty-fourth? Shame on you!"

She was looking at the food table. "I could have ice cream now?"

I just had to let it go, with all those people around us.

But later, I did have a T-shirt in her size printed up. It said in large letters on the back, "My birthday is March 24th."

She wore it to parties until she figured out what it said.

Over the years, she has been sung to in restaurants probably once a month. She finds a way to alert the waiter in the split second when we are not paying attention. We are totally surprised when the waiter brings a cupcake with a candle in it. If all her fake birthdays were real, she'd now be about five hundred years old.

Meanwhile, our Bammy was dying. Her cancer had spread. Mom, weak as she was, refused to put Bam in a nursing home and changed the soiled sheets on her bed twice a day. Finally Bam was hospitalized, and Mom and I sat at her bedside while she wrote us notes telling us to go home and get on with our lives. She had a tube in her throat and could not talk after her latest surgery.

A few weeks earlier, I had said to her, "Bammy, when I get to this point in my life I will not be able to take the suffering you're going through. I will find a way to do myself in."

She smiled at me and said, "Wait till you get here. You'll see you'll cling to life with all the strength you have. Now get me the newspaper and let's look at the brides and see which is the ugliest."

The days in the hospital wore on. Although she was mostly sound asleep, Bammy indeed was clinging. Mother sighed and said, "You have no idea how long it takes to get dead."

One morning while she was awake, Bammy wrote a note saying, "You be sure I'm dead." Mother read it, patted Bam's hand, smiled, and turned to tell me, "When she was a little girl, Bam heard a story about grave robbers digging up a grave. When they opened the wooden coffin, there were scratch marks on the lid and splinters under the fingernails of the dead man. He had woken up in his coffin and clawed it." She looked at Bam and said, "It's haunted you all your life, hasn't it, Bam?" She nodded.

Irene Armstrong Brainerd, whom I had tried to call Grammy but it came out Bammy when I was a baby, finally closed her eyes for the last time. She had built the little house on J Street as a widow, and then, being too lonely, begged my parents to buy it from her and let her live with them. She had been housekeeper, cook, and loving grandmother to Irene and me all our lives. No matter how you are expecting it, it's still such a loss when you have been loved the way Bam loved us. Sometimes people tell me they marvel at how kind and loving I am to my sister. The old saying "As you're done to, you will do" seems right on to me. When that kind of love is passed to you in a family, you pass it on. The nurturing, the caring, the kindnesses come naturally to you, because that's all you've known.

Irene had come to see Bammy in the hospital several times, and when it was over and we were planning the funeral, we remembered that Bam had once dreamed that at her funeral we danced in the aisles to "Alexander's Ragtime Band." It had made her so mad that she wouldn't speak to us for hours.

When we began humming it and then singing it, Irene brightened. "We could play that for Bammy?"

No. We couldn't.

We weren't into being haunted.

Eviction, Again

Irene got along fine in her apartment for a few years with Debbie, but when Debbie finished her degree, she had to move on. We hired another companion, who never cleaned the apartment, so we let her go. Then we hired another, who gave Irene her meals on the floor. When I dropped in one evening and saw this scene,

I told this companion that Irene was not a dog, and we let that companion go, too.

Finally we found the woman of our dreams: a single, middle-aged woman named Dana, who'd just returned from a Mormon mission to China. She loved Irene from the moment she met her. She had the main ingredients we needed: kindness and compassion and good cheer.

It did not go perfectly, but Dana learned quickly. For example, she immediately changed the décor of Irene's apartment: no glass on picture frames, and pretty baskets on the walls, since they don't injure people or property when being hurled about the room.

Irene went to Columbus Community Center during the day and took the bus home to Dana, who had nutritious meals waiting for her. The meals were even served at a table! Dana and Irene had beauty rituals together: coloring each other's hair or doing manicures and pedicures. They were real buddies. Despite Irene's periodic tantrums, which alarmed the neighbors, Dana and Irene managed for three years at that place, until the day they were evicted. And it turned out to be my fault.

Irene was already on probation with the manager of the apartment because of her tantrums. The neighbors could hear her through the walls, and the manager had called to warn us that one more infraction and it would be over. One day Dana called me to tell me Irene was having a real doozie. I could hear it in the background. Furniture was being turned over, the screaming was nonstop, and I heard her elbow go through a window, one of her favorite drama tricks.

Well, I had had it. "I'm on my way, Dana," I said.

Forget behavior mod techniques. Forget ignoring bad behavior. I had had it. This was going to change Irene's behavior once and for all.

When I got there, I barged in and launched into my routine. I was going to outdramatize her. Grabbing a newspaper and rolling it up and screaming at the top of my lungs, I pushed her down on her bed and whapped my open hand with the paper, yelling that I'd be damned if I'd stand for any more of this. A rolled-up newspaper makes an impressive noise.

Looking back on it, I wonder why I chose to forget the behavior lessons of Glenn Latham's about this. "If you yourself resort to yelling and hitting, you have lost the ball game. You are dead meat. The kid has won."

But would I recall this? No. After a minute or two of screaming and hitting my hand, the headboard, and the bed, I was getting hoarse, and it was a real effort to keep up the drama. I was using all my skills as an actress. I wasn't proud of my performance: yelling at your mentally disabled sibling is not ever one's finest hour, but there isn't a sibling in the world who hasn't been tempted. And she had driven me to this.

Was I noticing—no, it couldn't be—a slight smile on her face?

And then I realized: she had won again. All she wanted was more attention. Negative or positive didn't matter. Look what she had achieved: I had driven all the way out to her apartment, and she had my full attention. She was enjoying every minute of it.

To top it all off, the neighbors called the main office, saying they were trying to be kind and withstand Irene's tantrums, but now her *sister* was having them. They requested we all be removed permanently from the property. Eviction is such an ugly word, don't you think?

There used to be a sign on the bulletin board at the Texas offices of the National Association for Retarded Citizens. It said, "Starting over builds character." I copied it and put it on my desk, too.

Okay, I said, back to the drawing board. Irene needs a freestanding house, with fairly thick walls, so neighbors won't hear her screams when she decides to have a tantrum. I found a cute little brick bungalow for rent, and we tried that. Of course this would be the answer for Irene's life.

Once they realized that this grown woman wanted them to talk to her dolls, the neighbor children taunted her and made fun of her. On top of all that, Dana had to put a chain and padlock on the fridge, because she had heard Irene rooting around in it at three in the morning and found her eating frozen, raw chicken.

But Irene's situation had to wait. Mom and Dad, their health declining at an alarming rate, sold their lovely home and bought a condominium in a building right next to the one they had started their marriage in, sixty years before.

Their little apartment was perfect for them. The bay window overlooked the elegant fountain on the grounds near the Salt Lake LDS temple. Their balcony was lined with window boxes, so they could still plant tulip bulbs in anticipation of another spring. Meanwhile, Dad's lungs were giving out. I would visit him and pound his back for him. With people with emphysema, you have to pound their backs with the outer edges of your hands, whack, whack, whack, for a long time, to loosen the phlegm that builds up in their lungs.

"I have this idea about Irene," he said, his voice sounding

battered through my pummeling. "I know it may be impossible, but in the long run I envision her living in a neighborhood in her own place, being able to take the bus downtown, go shopping, take in a movie, and live like a normal, retired lady."

"Dad, that's almost what we have now. The neighbors are not as kind as we'd like, but eventually I can find a neighborhood that would work for her. Everything's going to be all right, really."

"Righto, Albert," he said.

I stopped whacking him. He lay back on his bed and said, "Did you hear Paul Harvey's broadcast today?" I shook my head no. And then he told me Harvey's ending story for the day.

Man goes into supermarket with a two-year-old boy, puts the boy in the grocery cart, and begins his shopping. The boy begins to yell and throw things out of the cart onto the floor. "Listen, Albert," the man says, "this will be over very soon. We just have to get a few items and then we'll be out of here, okay?" The boy continues misbehaving, throwing cereal boxes out of the shelves onto the floor, grabbing cans and throwing them, yelling all the while. Again the man says, "Everything's going to be all right, Albert." Finally they get up to checkout, and the little boy hurls all the mints and chewing gum to the floor. "Albert, we're going to be out of here and in the nice car in just a few minutes now! You can make it! Everything is going to be all right, Albert."

Finally a woman behind him says, "Sir, we've all been watching you with this boy. Your patience is just amazing. Little Albert is so lucky to have you for a father!"

The man looks startled and replies, "But, madam. *I* am Albert."

Dad and I cracked up. His laughter started a coughing fit that took a long time to calm down. I could see he was really in pain, and so very tired.

When he could talk again, he said, "Listen, honey. I may need you to do me a favor." He pulled out the drawer near his lounge chair. It was filled with vials of Mom's morphine. "I am going to have to get myself out of here soon. I can't stand struggling for breath every minute. I really want it to be over. I have these things at the ready, and may inject myself this week. But the damnedest thing is, I'm afraid I'll shake so hard that I'll botch the job. I want to be able to call you and have you come finish it."

"Oh, Dad, I know how much you need to get out. But that's murder! I would be put in prison for it."

"They'd never have to know."

"Dad. *I'd* know." I knew I could never do it, and I knew for sure then that we need to have a legal way to get out of this world ourselves if we're in that much pain and it's the end of our life anyway.

He just sighed and looked at me, as if I had failed him. "You'll whack me every day to keep me alive, when all I really want is for you to whack me once and for all?"

"But you don't want to leave Mom."

"Of course I don't. But you can't image how strong she really is, even in her condition. I think Bam and I have done her a disservice over the years. Since I've been so darned sick, she has climbed on a step stool and hammered nails in the wall to hang a picture. She gets her breakfast and mine every morning. She seems stronger every day!"

"Well, okay then. Now Dad, you do me a favor. If there is any way of your contacting me from the other side after you die, will you please do it?"

"Okay. I frankly think everything just goes black, but if I'm wrong and you're right, I'll do what I can."

"I just have this sense that there is something over on the other side, and that you will hang around me, at least for a while. So promise me."

He smiled. "I promise."

"Sorry about not being able to whack you for good."

"Me too."

But just two days later, on a Sunday, Mom called. "Terrell, come quick. I think your father's dying. I called 911 and they're on their way up, but meet us at the hospital, will you?"

Sure enough, Dad died two hours later in the emergency room. Irene came there, held Dad's hand, and told him she loved him. She was calm and hugged Mom, and then said she wanted to go back to her place. She was totally grown-up about it all. Go figure!

When I took Mom back to their apartment, I went straight to the drawer he had shown me. All the morphine was still in place. Nature, God bless her, had just finally taken her course.

Dad was seventy-eight, and a class act to the very end. I admired him more than anyone in my life. I think he could have been a fine novelist, but he chose instead to use his talent in advertising, which was a lot more financially secure, so that he could be sure Irene would be cared for after he died. I will always miss getting his phone call on June 25th. "Only six more months to go! Start your shopping list!"

Irene gave the closing prayer at his funeral. "Heavenly Father, please say hi to my daddy in heaven. He might play bridge with Bammy! Name of Jesus Christ, Amen."

Hell in Hawaii

Right after Dad's funeral, our traveling fitness group was planning to go to Hawaii. I was the exercise instructor for this group, and we had been taking vacations together for a number of years. In the depths of winter we would go to Mexico or Hawaii and dance on the beach for a week. We called ourselves the Silver Door. Twenty women usually went, and this trip was no exception. I felt I couldn't leave Mom and Irene in their grief, so I invited them to join us. The ladies of the group all knew them both, loved Mom, and didn't seem to mind that I brought Irene. So off we went to the island of Maui.

Irene loved wading on the beach. I thought it would help heal her grief about losing Dad. But I wasn't prepared for an incident that happened midweek.

Mom said she was going to go look around the clothing shops in the hotel. Now, another of Irene's behavior triggers is that she wants all shopping to be done for her exclusively. So she responded to Mom's plan by screaming. Here was a shopping trip, and she wasn't going to get any loot. She screamed so loudly that finally we heard a knock on our door. It was the hotel manager. "What is happening?" he asked.

Irene continued to scream and hit herself in the face.

The manager watched this drama and said, "I had complaints from other guests. They were afraid someone was being murdered."

He could see Irene was doing the whole show herself. "I can't allow this in the hotel," he said.

"I understand," I said. "It will stop very soon now." We were one scream away from being shown the door.

In a few minutes, Irene exhausted herself. Mom and I held our breath the rest of the week, being grateful that any outbursts Irene had were on the beach and not in the hotel. We hit rock bottom when she started pummeling me on the plane home. That did it. I feared for her companion Dana. So two weeks later, I put Irene in the Western Institute for Neuropsychiatry for a two-week evaluation. She was in a locked unit, under observation. This was in the days before the new miracle drugs had come out, so the diagnosis came back that drugs would not help her, that she was just spoiled, that we should fire Dana, the saint, because she let Irene get away with too much, and that Irene should enter a group home that specialized in behavior modification. That would shape her up.

I told them I was fairly well acquainted with such group homes, and that Irene had been expelled from that system years ago. Her social worker pointed out that much had happened since she was last their client, and they were now ready for her. She should enter one of the new group homes that had been established by one of the many residential programs now sprouting up all over the state. Could Irene's behavior change that much? If I didn't move her into a group home, would she finally start punching Dana? I couldn't allow that.

Her current living situation with Dana was the only program that hadn't evicted Irene, because I was in charge of it. Why should I put her back in with the "professionals" who said they could change her behavior? Was it doing her a service to leave her with Dana? How best to serve poor Dana, too?

So a few days later, I thought I'd just ask Irene herself about this. I keep forgetting that she cannot conceptualize an idea. We were sitting by the duck pond at Liberty Park, eating sandwiches, and Irene was gazing out over the water. "Irene," I said, "honey, I can help you get what you want, but you have to tell me. Listen to me first. Mom is too weak to have you living at home with her. Paul and I will be happy to have you stay with us now and then, but not to live with us every day. Anyway, you'd be bored living our life. You need to live your own life. You have to tell me. What is it that you really want?"

She gazed out at the pond, and I imagined her forming the words that would tell me her soul's secrets. Then she looked at me thoughtfully, and said, "I want—a hot dog."

9

Shall We Begin—Again?

So if you're up for ghost stories, I have to tell you this. Right after we got back from Hawaii, while Irene was being evaluated over at the institute, Paul and I were having our dinner in front of the television in our library. Shelves of books line the walls of this room. All of a sudden, a book made its way out of the bookshelf right above my head and fell on me. It really hurt. I rubbed my head and held the book. Paul had watched the whole thing, and all he could say was, "Jesus H. Christ!" How could one book make its way out of the shelf?

I looked at the book. It was a compilation of plays. The first one listed was *Berkeley Square* by John Balderston, about an American who goes to London and switches places with his ancestors of two centuries past. It was Dad's favorite play. I think he was trying to keep his promise to contact me if he possibly could. And time travel was his favorite subject. I would like to say here, for the record, in case certain ghosts are reading this, that it was a pretty clumsy gesture and the lump on the top of my head took two days to go down. Either Dad was telling me that he'd made contact, that time travel is possible, or maybe he was just telling me to go to London and stop trying to fix Irene. But Irene was due to get out of the institute in a few days. So I thanked Dad and put the book on a lower shelf.

Irene's evaluation, followed by recommendations from the professionals, showed me that I had been running a very strange and, frankly, stupid program. Poor Dana had never had any backups to give her time off. She had never had any training in behavior modification, which is now standard procedure. Irene controlled Dana with every trick she knew, and it wasn't helping Irene one bit. Her social worker encouraged me to apply to one of the behavior modification group homes. I did as she suggested. It would probably be the best thing for Irene, and that had to be my priority.

Looking back on it, all I really needed to do was get Dana into some good training and hire some backup help for her. It would have been a much smarter move. But, as usual, I listened to the professionals. After all, this is their business. And after all, these group homes all over the state, run by several different service providers, truly are a godsend to most families and to the men-tally disabled people who want their own independence. I kept hoping the system would work for Irene as well.

I am very grateful for professional advice, sometimes. I am glad the pros are around when I need them. My problem as Irene's sister is that I never know if my instincts are right or if I am nuts and the professionals are right. Usually it's about half and half, but I almost always guess the wrong half, too late.

So this time, I gave Dana her severance pay, turned in the key to the rental home, and enrolled Irene in one of the behavior modification group homes. I was lucky to get a spot, as they are in very high demand. Dana was very sad, as she simply loved Irene. I was too clueless to realize how important love is in the equation of caretaking.

When I told Irene that this was our new plan, she asked, "And I get to see Dana?"

"Sure. You can have visits together," I said. "But you're going to have house parents, who look really nice and fun."

"I could go out on a date with the guy?" she asked.

"Maybe."

Irene settled into a basement bedroom in the group home. The good part of it was that she didn't have a roommate to push around. But I could hardly wait to see what gimmick she'd pull to get out of there and get back home with Mom.

Her first trick was to get their attention by slamming doors. Irene can slam a door so hard it breaks the frame. She is very good at this, and it scares everyone. One time, in another setting, she slammed a door in a fit of temper. The force she used to slam the door cut off the tip of her thumb. It was a colorful night at the emergency room, with her staff carrying the tip of her thumb, in case they could reattach it. They could not.

Now, what the staff at the group home did about this behavior was to make Irene stand there and slam the door thirty-five times. They would not let her stop slamming the door. She got tired. They told her to keep slamming. It completely wore her out.

She never slammed a door again in that home. Mom and I were encouraged. The staff seemed to know their business. And they actually enjoyed Irene.

Their favorite incident happened when she was to take a taxi to our house for dinner one evening. She climbed into the cab and gave the driver a note with my address written on it. He squinted at it and said to her, "I can't read this handwriting."

This sent her into a frantic fit. She began to scream and hit her cheek. The cab driver was so terrified he got out of his cab and ran down the street. The staff, watching out the window, ran out and told him Irene was harmless, but they had to stop laughing first.

It turned out that the housefather, Don, did indeed take Irene on outings, which she considered real dates. The promise of an outing with Don meant perfect behavior for at least a couple of days. "I have a boyfriend," she giggled. "His name is Don."

"But what about Joy, his wife?" we'd ask her.

"They're just good friends."

The Bus Terminal Blues

It was during this time that we wanted Irene to take the bus from Columbus into town to meet me so that she could come to dinner at Mom's. I told her I'd meet her at the bus and drive her the rest of the way. When the bus came, she wasn't on it. When the next bus came, she wasn't on it. An hour had gone by. I was getting really worried.

I went to a phone booth and called the bus company and told them the problem. "Don't worry, we'll find her," they told me. "Meanwhile, come on over a couple of blocks to the bus terminal. It's where we sort everything out."

Arriving at the terminal, I saw lots of people sitting in the waiting room, and a line for the phone booth. The supervisor at the desk welcomed me and told me to describe Irene, and which bus she was expected to be on, and then she got on her phone to the bus drivers. I was really impressed. She told me to take a seat, and when news of Irene came, she would let me know.

I thought of someone kidnapping her. Then I remembered the O. Henry story, "The Ransom of Red Chief," about thugs who capture a little boy who is such a holy terror that that family charges the thugs a huge sum to take the kid back.

And I relaxed. I could take that tack if necessary.

The local bus terminal was one block from the Greyhound terminal, so people were coming in from all around the country and then trying to make a local connection here. When I stopped fussing about losing Irene, I began to observe these travelers all around me. I overheard an African American man in the phone booth. He looked poor and hungry. "Hi, Ida," he said hopefully into the phone. "It's Tom. Yeah. Well, I was just passing through and thought I'd give you a call, maybe come see you—" Then silence. "Uh-huh. Okay. Sure. I see. Well, maybe another time . . ." and he hung up. He made three other calls like this, and with each call my perspective became a little sharper about what sadness is. What loneliness is. What total helplessness is. The man hung the phone up after his third call and walked, dejected, out of the terminal. I wanted to go give him money, but I thought it might humiliate him.

Then I saw a woman pick up the phone. "It's me, Ben. I'm leaving and don't try to come after me. No, goddamn you, I've had it. Oh, shut up. I'm out of here. For good, you bastard!" She slammed the phone back in its cradle, picked up her battered suitcase, and hurried out to board a bus. Other people sat there, staring ahead, with whatever loneliness and alienation they appeared to be feeling. I was one with them, for about a half hour. I had all the resources in the world. I knew everyone in town. Hell,

I could call the governor if I wanted! But no amount of influence or resources could help me now. My sister was lost, and not even the governor could do much about it. We all sat there, staring out the window, wondering how to solve our messy lives.

I was very close to standing up and announcing, "Okay, as soon as I find my sister, you're all coming home to dinner with me."

But I restrained myself. They'd think I was nuts. And maybe they had other plans. Soon a bus appeared, its only passenger being my sister. She hopped off the bus absolutely delighted that I was there. "I took the wrong bus!" she announced sheepishly, grinning from ear to ear.

"I sort of figured that out," I said, hugging her, and we went on our way, Irene thrilled to be rescued and me deeply grateful to have somewhere to go, to someone who loved us, to a warm home.

Irene's group home situation was not working out, surprise, surprise. Even though her staff told the spooked cab driver that she was completely harmless, that wasn't precisely accurate. When she slugged her housemates for the fourth time, it came to the staff's attention that she needed her own space, so they moved her to a semi-independent apartment, where she had the whole place to herself. Staff checked on her before and after her workshop job, and took shifts to be with her on weekends. That, they said, was all the supervision she really needed.

"Really?" I said. "Just a little checking in now and then? She needs no more help than that, huh?"

"That's right," said the supervised apartment living director, who maybe needed to fill his quota of clients to make budget for that quarter. "She'll do just fine here."

Uh-huh. Oh, yeah.

10

Travels with Mom

"Terrell, leave it to the pros. Irene will be fine," my friends with siblings or children in the group homes told me. "Really, the staff is terrific, and she will be with her peers, so stop fussing! Give it a few months. See how it turns out."

Meanwhile Mom said, "I want to go on a last trip. I'd like to take you on a cruise in the Mediterranean, and we'll stop in New York on the way home and see some shows. That's what I want." She sighed. "It will be my very last trip to New York."

So what's not to like about a cruise in the Mediterranean? I told Mom of course I would go.

On the ship-to-shore excursions, Mom had organized taxis to take us to places she and Dad had loved. One gorgeous autumn afternoon in Venice, we took a water taxi to the dock by the Hotel Danieli and had lunch in its rooftop restaurant overlooking the Grand Canal. As we clinked our wine glasses and saluted each other, I thought to myself, here I am in the most romantic spot on earth—with my mother. It was an unkind thought, especially since after lunch she limped her way into San Marco Square to take me to a little shop she recalled that sold jewelry made out of Venetian glass crystals. She bought me earrings, a necklace, and a bracelet, and I realized, as we made our way back to the water taxi and the ship, what an ungrateful wretch I was.

But here's the rub of the trip for me: I was exhausted from caretaking. By now Mom needed a wheelchair in airports and for long walks, and I pushed her, along with all the other caretakers I saw on the cruise ship, all in exactly the same boat (pardon the pun) as I was.

At night, when we had got our charges to bed, we walked the ship, we caretakers. There must have been at least thirty of us: hired help or the grandchildren or spouses of those who were too weak to travel but still wanted to go. I looked at us all, strolling along the deck, and it occurred to me that we paid a fairly heavy price for our good health, in a way. I was so tired that the thought of someone pushing *me* in a wheelchair and bringing me breakfast in bed sounded wonderful. The other caregivers looked equally haggard. We didn't speak. The quiet of the night felt wonderful. It was our only time to be alone with our own thoughts.

One night our Greek cabin steward whispered to me, "Meet me in the hall, please." He had been watching me wait on Mom for a week. In the hall, he said, "You need to have more fun on this cruise. When your mother is all settled for the night, tell her the crew has invited you to a party below."

I did. Mom said, "Have a good time, dear," and off I went into the bowels of the ship with my cabin steward, where the wine was flowing and the Greek music was playing. I found myself immediately pulled into a circle of Greek dancing, Zorba style. We danced until one in the morning, and my exhaustion fell away with all the music and camaraderie of the delightful crew, men and women of all ages, just letting loose. As I crawled into bed, I thought to myself, yes, there's a price for caretaking, but now and then it has its rewards. If that cabin steward had considered me just another privileged passenger, he would never have invited me. I got a pass to the crew party because I was a worker, just like them.

Back in New York, checking into the Marriott, I try my usual con game again. "This is my mother's very last trip to New York, and I was wondering if we could have a room with a nice view." The clerk looks at me and then at Mother, "Just one minute, ma'am," he says, clicking his computer and staring at the screen.

It works.

Mom is thrilled with the view, even though her eyes now make fuzzy stars of each point of light. ("Don't worry," she has told me. "It just makes things doubly glamorous.") As I start to unpack and turn down her bed, she says, "No, not yet. I've heard they have a wonderful bar here that rotates around slowly so you can see the whole skyline. Let's go up and have a nightcap!"

I am exhausted and achy, seeing my life stretch out as perpetual caretaker not only for Irene but also for my mom, who has been dying on my arm for the last five years and is planning on five years more.

"Okay! Let's do it!" I say brightly, smiling. I hate phony people, yet at times, I am the biggest phony I know.

Half an hour later we are seated at the window of The View with two big manhattans. "Isn't this lovely! And aren't we lucky to be able to be here! Let's be sure to send Irene a postcard." She lifts her glass for a toast, her hand shaking so badly the drink almost spills. At this point she has cancer, heart disease, ulcers from radiation treatments, osteoporosis, familial tremor in her hands, and cataracts in her eyes. She considers all these minor inconveniences that must be overcome on the way to the theater—any theater, anytime, anywhere. If someone is standing on a stage doing almost anything, Mom wants to be there, clapping.

When I was in grade school, Mother would come and take me out for an afternoon matinee if a touring company of any Broadway play was in town. "But," the teacher would say, "school isn't out until three thirty."

"Oh, I know," she'd say, "but this is *the theater.* We have a matinee, and you know they always begin at two." She was surprised that the teacher didn't know that going to a play or a musical should take precedence over everything.

One year she had a heart attack and insisted on leaving the hospital three days early because she had tickets to the road company production of *The Unsinkable Molly Brown.*

"Let's see, now, what's our matinee tomorrow?" she asks.

"*Guys and Dolls,*" I tell her, waiting now for the familiar recital of how no one could ever do Adelaide like Vivian Blaine did. I get it. I sip my manhattan and listen again, and I know what's coming next: the failings of theater today compared to theater in *her* day. She watched the curtain rise on Lynn Fontanne in *O Mistress Mine.* "The set dazzled the audience. It was a gorgeous drawing room. Lynn Fontanne sat there on a green velvet love seat. She was dressed in ruby red satin with a flowing skirt, a huge vase of ruby red roses on the table behind her. The audience just gasped and began to applaud, and she had to wait about three minutes until the clapping died down to say her first line."

She also had the fun of watching Alfred Drake stroll onstage to sing about a bright golden haze on the meadow, the opening song in *Okalahoma,* which she now proceeds to tell me about again. I am both envious of her having those early Broadway nights and exhausted from hearing about them for the fiftieth time. She brought the record albums home from each trip, and as a child, I would dance and sing to them in the living room.

"Did I tell you about Gertrude Lawrence in *Skylark?*" Now *there* was a play." Which is now going to segue into seeing Gertie do *The King and I.* Knowing the entire script, I take another swig of my cocktail and wonder how I can beg a cab driver to drive us just one block to lunch at Sardi's tomorrow.

How can she still be upright? Can passion for the theater translate into sheer will and win over a failing body? I listen and drink until the lights of Manhattan look fuzzy to me, too. I wonder if I will do this to my girls: tell them my memories over and over. Will they have to almost carry me to the theater? I think of an old Spanish proverb: Ill women never die. Is this my genetic heritage?

"Well, that was perfect," she says, having finished her monologue on People Who Could Not Sing But Did The Part Anyway, like Gertrude Lawrence, and then her dearest love, Rex Harrison, in *My Fair Lady.* "Let's go to bed now. But I do love the idea that these actors used their best skills, acting, and just overlooked their weaknesses. It's like playing a hand of bridge. You work with what you've got." I pay the bill and manage to pull her to her feet.

It takes a half hour to get back to our room, she moves so slowly. Lowering Mom into the hot bath, I picture her lowering me into our tub on J Street when I was a year old. It's all in the home movies. Now Mom's body looks as bad as any prisoner from the World War II photos: flesh with purple sores hanging on protruding bone. *"Guys and Dolls,"* she says happily. "The opening song, about a horse right here, always ends in 'can do.' I love that. It's really how I've tried to live my life. Now hand me a washcloth, darling."

Sardi's comforts Mom. She goes to this restaurant to be back in the 1940s. She is telling me the story of her grandmother auditioning for a part on the stage. "She got a call-back, and was so excited, and went home to tell her father about it. He told her ladies did not act on the stage and forbade her to go back. She was heartsick, but she stayed home like a good girl."

In fact, Mom and Dad met for the first time on the stage at the East High senior production of *Pocahontas*. She played an Indian maiden and Dad was a stagehand. As the curtain came down during rehearsal, she was standing right where the curtain would hit her on the head. My father grabbed her shoulders and shoved her out of the way, where she promptly fell down. After picking her up and apologizing, he asked her out the next day.

There's the whole story of our family, I thought. Stagestruck wannabees. Mom is gazing at the pictures on the wall. "You could have been up there," she says.

"Doing what?" I ask.

"Oh, as the playwright. Or the actress or singer."

"Mom. I have spent my life staying home, just like my great-grandmother and grandmother and you. I did community service and had little paid jobettes, not a career. They don't put pictures of us on the wall at Sardi's."

She chews her cannelloni. "Well, maybe they ought to."

Getting a cab after a matinee with Mother in tow requires

beating out other old ladies only slightly less frail. It always works, but it takes everything out of me. Once settled in the cab, I have to tell the driver, "The Marriott Marquis, please."

"Lady, it's right there," he says, pointing one block ahead.

"I know. But my mother can't walk that far."

The cab driver sighs and we lurch forward. It's hard to say this, because inside this frail little woman is the strongest human being I've ever known. She has shrunk to the size of all the Japanese tourists flooding the halls of the Marriott, but I think she could whip them all in a fight. My back is killing me from hefting Mother, hefting suitcases, grabbing cabs. It will take me a week to recuperate, but Mom is simply glowing. As usual, she's just playing from the strong cards in her hand. After all, she points out to me, this is her Very Last Trip to New York.

11

Losses and Tantrums (Mine)

Still trusting the group home and sheltered-workshop system, I visited Irene at her apartment occasionally and had her to family dinners and birthday celebrations. I was still worried about her situation, as she was gaining weight steadily and did not look all that happy, but I was busy with our family.

Our daughters Katy and Marriott had each found superb men to marry: John for Katy, Craig for Marriott—men Paul and I can hardly stand to call sons-in-law because they feel like our own sons. We had two weddings two years apart, and Irene was in charge of the guest book for each wedding.

Later on, when my elder daughter, Kate, became pregnant, Mom could hardly wait to meet her great-grandchild, due in February.

On the second day of December, almost three months before Katy's delivery day, I called Mom. Our plan was to get her Christmas tree that day. "You know, honey," she said, "it's so cold out, I don't want to look all over the lot for a tree. Will you go pick one out, you know the kind I like, and I'll just walk to the Alta Club for my lunch and bridge game."

"Mom, it's cold enough out that I ought to come drive you over there."

"Half a block? That's ridiculous! I'm fine, and I can walk home, too. Gaylie (her best friend) will walk me down the stairs at the end of the afternoon."

"I'm afraid you'll fall."

"Well, don't be. Every time I fall, I keep thinking to myself, 'Well, good. This is it, I'll be dead now,' but I never quite fall hard enough! It's very vexing, because that is a perfect way to get out of here: just, you know, boom, it's over. So don't worry about that. Worry that I won't fall hard enough!"

So I went shopping for her Christmas tree. I found a perfect one for her, blue spruce with lots of room between the branches so that her gorgeous angels and crystal ornaments would show off well. I was just pulling into my own garage, planning to unload my groceries and then go down to deliver Mom's tree, when Paul called. "Where have you been? I've been trying to reach you for an hour. Your mom fell on the steps of the Alta Club and is still unconscious. I'm at LDS emergency room. Come over."

The doctor greeted me and told me, "She's on life support. The machine is breathing for her, but that fall was so hard she is brain-dead. I can keep her alive like this, but she could remain in a coma forever. I don't think she'll regain consciousness. If it were my mother, I would let her go."

Mom's friend Gaylie later told me that she was helping her down the stairs. There was no ice on the stairs. Mom suddenly pulled away from her, as if she were being pushed by an unseen hand, and fell, hitting the back of her head so hard that the medical examiner had to look at her to make sure she had not been murdered with an axe. Gaylie said, "Terrell, I wonder if your father's spirit came along and pushed her, hard. That's exactly what it felt like. I couldn't grab her to help her, she went down so hard and fast." Just as Mom had said to me that morning, "Worry that I won't fall hard enough." She got her wish.

I called Irene and had one of her companions bring her to the hospital. She wept with me, held Mom's hand, and understood. Please, Lord, tell me, how can Irene go through these huge crises of our parents' and Bammy's deaths with quiet dignity and then scream when someone touches her purse or her doll?

Uncle Bob, Mom's brother, came. We sat by her bed for a long time. Then, together, we let Mom go. We knew that, in her soul, she was cheering. It was time.

Irene asked if she could stay with me for a couple of days—she felt so lonely out at her apartment. I went out and picked her up, telling her staff she needed to be with family. But when it came time to go to the funeral home and choose a coffin, I didn't think she'd be able to handle that. So I called Uncle Bob and asked him if he could take Irene for an hour. "Hell, Tiger. What would I do with her?" (One hour, Bob? Just one hour? I was stunned that he wouldn't help me.)

"Okay. Never mind," I said. I didn't even think of asking my girls to take her. It had been my habit not to bother them with Irene except for family functions where I would be there to supervise her. So I took Irene along with me. It turned out she did just fine with coffins.

What she kept asking me was if she could please have Mom's apartment and live there. On the face of it, this seemed like a reasonable solution for her. But the place wasn't configured well for a staff member to care for her there, and downstairs on the first floor sat Irene's idea of heaven: a little Quickie Mart, chock full of deli items, soda pop, and potato chips. She would try to live in that store and drive everyone nuts. I had to tell her we couldn't afford for her to stay in Mom's apartment; I needed to sell it and put the money in trust for her, and maybe we could find something else, not so expensive. I was exhausted, and felt so guilty that I started to cry about not being able to let her stay there. She put her arm around me and said, "That's okay, Terrell. I like the money too."

At Mom's funeral, after my daughters and I spoke about Mom's life, and Irene said a very gracious closing prayer, we asked the audience to feel free to stand up and tell any stories about Mom they wanted to share. Her friend Blanche Freed, who had been playing at that last bridge game at the Alta Club, said, "You know, I went to school with Afton and Dick. Dick's mother had me all picked out for Dick, and then he met Afton! Well, she got that lovely man, and I got . . ." She turned to look down at her husband, sitting there next to her. She looked as if she had got tenth prize. "I got David here."

When everyone stopped laughing, she went on. "Afton Harris went out of here in the best and fastest way possible. I so envy that. And to top it all off, she won the pot that day in our bridge game!"

When I went to Mom's condo to go through her immaculate closet, there was her black fox fur muff that she'd had since the 1940s. I buried my nose in it, trying to inhale some of my childhood: that elegant smell of Joy perfume and fresh violets that always surrounded her.

I pictured her as a child herself, in her dress and hat and

patent leather shoes, skipping along with friends, playing with her dolls, feeling full of love and hope for her own future. I pictured the terrible disease of rheumatoid arthritis invading her just after her eighteenth birthday, while she was sailing to Europe on a tour with her girlfriends. I pictured all the pain she had experienced, and the crippling of her hands and knees and feet. I pictured the agony of Irene's birth, and the constant challenge of dealing with her own physical pain while trying to cope with Irene. And I pictured her sitting under the tree at the Wasatch Riding Academy, reading her novel, making sure her elder child got to live her fondest dreams, too. It just came crashing in on me how Mom had done her level best for both her children. I looked at the neatly folded panty hose in her drawer, along with her beautiful white leather gloves, saved in hopes they'd come back into style. How did she get those panty hose on every day, when her hands wouldn't work, and her knees wouldn't bend? How did she even face every day?

Oh, Mom. How can you forgive me for not understanding you more?

You can really mess up a fur muff with tears and a runny nose.

To this day, Mom is with me. Whenever I wrap a package, I remember her elegant boxes with lovingly tied ribbons, and I hear her voice: "Put that little flower through the ribbon there. That makes it fancier. Tie a candy cane into that bow; it goes with the wrapping."

But her main trademark in life was making every person she met feel special and important, from her bridge friends to the lady who cleaned her house. Every day she headed to lunch with her friends, played bridge like a champion, and never complained about her pain. Now and then she would go to our city's fabulous candy store, Cummings Candy, and buy chocolates to take to the nursing home where Bammy's friends still lived and played bridge.

When I think of all of us trying for our version of a successful life, which nowadays seems to mean being very rich and very famous, I think of Mom limping into a nursing home to deliver those chocolates to a dear and aging friend, and I think I know what a truly successful life might look like. She made everyone she met feel welcome, as if she were honored to be in their company.

The line to get into her funeral went halfway around the block, and standing in it were old friends, their children, waitresses from her clubs, women who were in her Brownie troop as children. It seemed to include everyone who had ever met her. Talk about a class act.

I Have My Own Tantrum (Again)

Mom's death had now left me with three things: a medium-sized inheritance that could be applied toward Irene's improved well-being; a big concern that I wasn't giving her the life that Dad had described to me before he died; and a truckload of guilt for having a nice life, a nice home, and a loving family all around me.

So I turned into a carping fool. A few days after Mom's funeral, I went out to visit Irene in her latest supervised apartment, across town. I had tried to ignore the messiness when I went to visit her. Normal people are not all neatniks, I told myself, remembering my teenagers' rooms. Relax. Let it go. Let her have her own life and experience. I had been telling myself that for about five years while she lived in one supervised apartment after another.

But this day I had bought her some new underwear, and as I was putting it in her drawer, I noticed that all the other clothes in the drawer were damp.

I went into the front room, and there her staff member sat, watching her favorite TV show. I held out a pair of damp pajama tops. "Sherry. Honey. Come feel this," I said. Sherry, who looked about seventeen and very pregnant, dutifully rose from the couch and came to feel the damp top. "What's wrong?"

"They're wet," I said, staring at her. "They were in her drawer. They were never dried in the dryer."

"Oh," she said, staring back at me. "Well, it didn't happen on my shift."

As long as Sherry was up off the couch, I took the opportunity to take her into the kitchen, where dishes were piled up and pizza boxes were spilling out of week-old garbage. "Is this the way you think the kitchen should look?" I ask her.

She said, "Well, see, Irene's supposed to do this stuff herself."

Irene was taking a bath at the time, so I felt perfectly comfortable telling Sherry what I thought, straight out. "Listen, Sherry. Irene is not lazy and spoiled. She is mentally disabled."

"We call it special needs now."

"Call it what you want, sweetheart. She doesn't know how long clothes are supposed to dry, and she will never get her dishes right or take out her own garbage because she doesn't even care if it's piling up! She is fifty-five years old, she won't wear her glasses, and she can't see the dishes well enough to rinse them, so they go in the dishwasher caked with food that doesn't come off. She needs more help than you guys are giving her."

Sherry, whose paycheck was less than she could make at McDonald's, looked at me and said, "They taught us in training not to do their work for them. When they're in a supervised apartment like this, they're supposed to do all their own work."

"I see. So your job, then, is to sit on the couch and watch your favorite shows for your shift?" I felt sorry for Sherry, but sorrier for Irene.

Sherry leaned from one foot to the other. "Do you want to call my supervisor? She'll explain the program to you."

All I needed was to have the program explained to me. My heart was pounding with anger. "Good. Let's just give her a call, shall we?"

I felt I was familiar enough with the rules to have a little chat with the supervisor. Fifteen minutes later she showed up—a woman whom I'll call Michelle. Irene was out of the bathtub now and in her pajamas—some dry ones, not the wet ones—and listening intently to my exchange with Michelle.

"I would like for you to explain to me what the job of this staff is," I said to Michele.

"Their job is to make sure these people have the least restrictive alternative to a normal life, and to assist them in becoming even more independent."

"Don't give me the bureaucratic gobbledygook," I said, "because I wrote it. Just tell me how a filthy kitchen and wet laundry fit into this scenario."

She narrowed her eyes. "When Irene is tired of dirty dishes and wet laundry, she'll do them right," she said.

"So you're just letting her wallow in it until she's sick of it?"

"That's right. She's perfectly capable—"

"No, actually, she isn't. That's why she needs help."

"Well, we're not going to wait on her."

"How about a little assistance for her while she's trying to do it?"

"She wants us to do it all. She's spoiled."

"She is also a little disabled, have you noticed, Michelle?"

"She's not as disabled as you think."

"Okay. Call her Superwoman. But yesterday I peeked in, and I found another of her helpers, Matt, the one with the cowboy boots, lying on her couch watching a football game, and yelling, 'Irene, go do your dishes.' She was standing there, asking Matt if she could see her favorite program, which is *ER,* and he was telling her, no, he was going to watch the game while she did her dishes."

Michelle stiffened and folded her arms. She opened her mouth to speak, but my cosmic anger and I were on a roll. "Is pizza all you guys ever get for dinner? Could someone please cook some fresh vegetables? My God, she's gaining weight—sorry, Irene, but you are—and I have to order her clothes from special catalogs because she's now a 5X and no one in town carries that size! Listen, your program is not as advertised, and believe me, not as originally designed. You can trust me on this."

Michelle stood up and narrowed her eyes even further. "What were you doing driving clear across town to check up on us, *two days in a row?* You know what you are? You are a raging codependent! My God, why don't you get a *life?*" And she stormed out of the apartment.

Sherry looked embarrassed as the door slammed, and said, "Listen, this job is harder than it looks. See, Irene doesn't wipe herself after going to the bathroom. I mean, yesterday morning, when I dropped Irene off at work, she was sliding on something on my car seat, and when I looked at it when she got up, I realized it was her own poop! My car still stinks!"

We stood there, staring at each other. I was horrified, for Sherry and for Irene. "Did you let her go into the workshop like that?"

"Well, yeah . . . it was the end of my shift and I had to go to my other job. . . ."

It took me a few minutes to absorb the reality that this was as good as this program is going to get, given the budget, the age of the staff, and staff turnover. These young people on the staff, good kids who wanted to make a contribution in the world rather than flip burgers for maybe fifty cents more, were all doing the best they could. And they didn't stay long in the job because it's hard and dirty and frustrating and they were getting paid very little. The good people who run the group homes hire the best talent they can find for the price. I knew they were doing their best, too. Many of their clients thrived in the program we had set up. Maybe Irene was thriving, in her own fashion, and I just got too picky, forgetting that nothing is perfect.

"Thanks, Sherry," I told her, "for telling me how it really is. I'm sorry to be so critical."

Sherry left. I did Irene's mountain of dishes while she watched me. I took out the garbage. She asked me for money. I felt sorry for her. I gave her two dollars. "Get quarters so you can do your laundry, okay?"

"Okay," she said, hugging me.

I learned later that after I left she went downstairs to the candy machine and had a very happy evening. A helper found the candy wrappings the next morning. And all the laundry in her drawers was still wet.

I lay awake all night. Many fine group home providers existed now, and Irene was in one of the best, as far as I knew, but it really didn't work for her, or for me. Did I have enough in the trust fund Dad and Mom left for her care that I could make it last all her life? How would it work if I moved her in with Paul and me? What if she outlived me?

I couldn't ask Paul to take her in permanently, although I know he would make the effort and help me until we found a better solution. In the morning, I told him my dilemma. "You can't fix everything every minute," he said. "Let Irene's life be *their* problem."

"The group home supervisor called me a raging codependent and told me to get a life," I told him.

"Well, sticks and stones," he yawned. "What is a codependent?"

"A person who needs to make everything all better for people, even when it's impossible."

"Hmm," he said. "The shoe really fits, doesn't it?"

"Oh shut up," I said, cuddling into his arms.

A week later, I got a letter from Michelle, apologizing for being critical of me and reaffirming that she really had Irene's best interests at heart. She wanted me to know that what I wanted for Irene's life was often not what Irene wanted. Also, what Irene wants, she pointed out, is usually not what she needs. She suggested that I had a hard time separating things and activities that I would like from things that Irene would like. She said if I could work on separating myself a little more from my sister, she—and I—might have happier lives in the long run, which was all the staff was trying to do for us.

I read the letter and stared out the window for a long time.

Of course, Michelle was right. I remembered the previous New Year's Eve, when I was going to a glamorous party and fussing that Irene had nothing to do on this festive night. Finally I bought tickets for First Night, our city celebration held downtown, with everything from jugglers to ballet performances. I sent them to Irene with the suggestion that one of her helpers could take her down there.

Well, it completely ruined her New Year's Eve. She did not want to go downtown in the crowds. She wanted to stay home with her helper, eat popcorn, drink fake champagne, watch a video, and see the ball drop in Times Square. But knowing I had a different plan for her, absolutely sure she would love it, she reluctantly bundled up and went with her helper to the car. Whereupon she began to hit herself over and over because she didn't want to be cold and crowded. The helper turned back toward home and Irene wailed, "No, Terrell wants me to go! I have to go! She'll be mad I didn't use the tickets!" After two hours of turning toward home and then turning back toward town, they finally got back and Irene fell into bed, swollen-faced and exhausted.

I pinned Michelle's letter to my bulletin board as a constant reminder to myself of how much I had yet to learn and how maybe I had abused her well-meaning staff. If I weren't so obsessed, I *could* leave Irene in the program across the city, trust the staff, and let her live her own life without so much help—or interference—from her sister. Surely they must be right and I must be a very sick person. This was my dark night of the soul. Michelle told me to get a life. But Irene was a part of that life. I didn't think Mom and Dad would like the way she was living.

12

Trying to Get a Life

I wanted to say to Michelle, listen, it isn't as if I don't *have* a life. I *have* a life. I've had many lives.

Looking back on my life, I realized that at Stanford, I was doing what young women did in the 1950s: looking for a suitable husband. The dean of women there said to me, "I hope you're not going to just give your life to a man and end up sorting his socks. Too many bright Stanford women end up spending their lives sorting some man's socks."

I had heard that she was unmarried, no doubt jealous of happy homemakers with families. So I ignored her completely, found a suitable husband, and landed in my laundry dungeon in the basement, sorting his socks and ruminating on how right she was, how Paul should sort his own damn socks, and how I really should be elsewhere, using my fine mind and God-given talents.

I wrote my weekly newspaper column, made the odd television commercial now and then, and nagged legislators about programs for the developmentally disabled—but I had no real career. While I folded laundry, I ruminated and fantasized about what I should really be doing that would be satisfying.

My favorite fantasies had to do with going on the stage. I just knew I would be terrific. I certainly nailed every role in my living room as a child, singing along with all Mom's Broadway record albums when everyone was out of the house. My dancing seemed quite fine to me, too.

One day I climbed up the stairs with a load of clean laundry and a new world opened up to me. A newspaper article on the hall table almost leapt from the page: Auditions Held for Local Productions. And there, before my very eyes, was the show, in capital letters: *GYPSY.* I put the laundry down, sat on the stairs, and read that auditions for all parts were being held in two days.

It never occurred to me that I could not be the lead in *Gypsy.* I was perfect for it! I hurled myself over to the theater and put my name on the audition list. Then I asked where I could find a piano player to help me. They gave me her name, and in two days we had worked up a little song. I had been in show business since I was three. I knew what I was doing. Okay, so it was only doing commercials and radio spots, but I knew I could do this.

When it came time to audition, I saw that the fellow doing the auditioning was my old pal Keith, who had been with me in about a hundred commercials from early television days. He saw how very much I wanted to be in this show. I sang my heart out. Keith said thank you, he'd call me. If there was a look of tragic pity on his face, I never noticed it. That night he called. "Listen, Terrell, we are using Sue Ane Langdon from L.A. for Mama Rose, but would you like to be the walk-through for her part until she gets here?" Then, he said, the director, Tony Tanner, would place me in the show in a role appropriate to my experience. I nearly died of joy.

After the first rehearsal, when Tony heard me sing, he took me aside and said, "Tell me something. Why would you, with your very limited stage experience, try for the most demanding role ever written for a woman on Broadway?"

I didn't realize that by the fourth song I would be hoarse, and by the seventh song my voice would be gone and I would be whispering. For Mama Rose, you need lungs the size of dirigibles and the stamina of a Marine. He also told me I was way too nice to be the fiery, fierce Mama Rose. Why I thought I could do it, I'll never know. But the director knew it, and when Miss Langdon arrived, he put me where I belonged. He let me be a Christmas tree, a waitress, and in my most memorable role, the back end of the cow. He also suggested I might want to take a singing lesson or two.

My daughter Marriott was a shepherdess in the first act, and two of her friends joined the cast as well. Every night of the three-week run I sat in my cow costume on the steps leading into the orchestra pit and listened to the best overture ever written. It was heaven. Everything was coming up roses for me, even though I didn't have quite the role I wanted.

I took the director's advice and took some singing lessons. When I practiced in my living room, our black cat, Chimneysweep, would come close to me, and when I hit a high note, she would bite my ankle to get me to stop. I never once took it as a hint about my talents. I just thought poor Chimneysweep had sensitive ears.

It was about this time that I got a volunteer offer I couldn't

refuse. Two young men had hatched an idea for a Utah film festival that would feature classic old films and have famous people
come and talk about them. A sidelight of the event would be to
invite independent filmmakers to show their work in a juried
competition. The third goal was to get more film companies to
make their movies in Utah. One of the young men was John Earl
of the Utah Film Commission. The other was filmmaker Sterling Van Wagenen, who was the cousin of Lola Van Wagenen,
Robert Redford's wife at the time. They had heard that I could
organize things pretty well, and that I might be a good person to
help them get started. They called me and introduced themselves, and then the conversation went like this.

"We want you to be on the board of the new Utah/US Film
Festival."

"Oh, listen, guys, thanks for thinking of me, but I really can't.
I'm way too busy."

"Well, then, Robert and Katharine will be really disappointed. We know they were eager to work with you."

"Robert and Katharine who?"

"Redford. And Ross."

Long silence. "Well, you know, maybe I can work around
some of my projects . . ."

Thus, indeed, is a sucker born every minute, and I was the one
that particular minute, hooked by my own star worship. "Okay,"
I told them later, when they announced that a real meeting was
taking place, and that Robert was there waiting, and Katharine
was flying in, "but I get to drive Katharine down to Sundance for
the meeting."

"Done!" they said.

I was dying to meet the gorgeous Katharine Ross. I called

her hotel room to tell her I was ready to drive her down to Sundance. "Oh, I'll be right there!" she said.

"Katharine?" I asked. "How will I know you?"

"Well, I'm in blue jeans and a maroon silk blouse . . ."

"Katharine," I said, "Just kidding."

She was so tiny she came up to my shoulder, and she was even more beautiful in real life. I asked her what she thought of this festival idea. She said she was just happy to be invited to Utah and go horseback riding with her friend Bob. She had certainly never heard of me or anyone else on the festival staff.

When we got to Sundance, we walked into the meeting, and Robert Redford jumped up to wrap his arms around her. Then they introduced him to me. He did not look thrilled to meet me or relieved that I had accepted the board position. In fact, when we all sat back down, he said, "Now what's this meeting about, anyway?"

They described to him the festival idea and its goals. "A film festival?" he said, ballpoint pen in hand, autographing one T-shirt after another, handed to him by his assistant, for some charity auction somewhere. "Don't have a film festival. They're a dime a dozen all over the world. If there's any project around film that should be done, it should be one I've been thinking about: having a sort of workshop, or institute, on the improvement of the whole industry. One week would be devoted to just lighting designers; one to just cinematography, one to set design, see what I mean? Maybe a week on scripts, or directing. Who's in charge of your festival thing?"

His cousin-in-law Sterling pushed the first Utah/US Film Festival program, already printed, thousands of copies, in front of him. It said, "Chairman: Robert Redford."

Redford was horrified. They told him, come on, you'll come to love it. It will be good for Utah, you'll see. He looked at us all around the table and then at the ceiling, probably counting to ten to calm himself. I just shook my head, wondering how I could let these people from Wonderland hook me in so easily by wanting to be around famous people.

In the long run, for me it was a bizarre and wonderful adventure. The second year of the festival, the awards banquet for independent films, which they asked me to emcee, actually drew Frank Capra, Jimmy Stewart, Robert Stack, and several other stars, in a tribute to Frank Capra's films.

Jimmy Stewart was the consummate pro. He and Frank Capra arrived and shook our hands, and then Jimmy said to me, "Okay, let's go strolling." He knew exactly why he was there: to have his picture taken with as many people as he could before dinner started, as a special perk for the $500 they paid per ticket. I escorted him around and watched. When people tried to hold onto him, he had the loveliest way of patting their hand on his arm and saying, "I'm strolling now. I know you understand," and they'd release their grip. At dinner he sat next to me, there at the Alta Club, where Paul and I had held our wedding reception. If Gene Autry was my big brush with the stars, hey, look at me now!

When it was my turn to announce the winners of the independent film competition, I had each filmmaker stand up while I read his credentials. The only thing was, I had the wrong credentials for each filmmaker. Each time a filmmaker stood up and I read his titles, he would shake his head. It got to be like an episode of *I Love Lucy*. The audience was hysterical, slapping their thighs, it was so funny. At the end of the nightmare, I just gave up on trying to match the right film with each filmmaker and had them speak for themselves. Jimmy Stewart came up to me and put his arms around me and hugged me for a long time, shaking with laughter. "Just thought I'd show you how we do things in Utah," I mumbled into his chest.

"You made my day," he said, kissing me on the top of my head.

I left the board the third year, when an angel by the name of Chuck Sellier donated $75,000 to get us out of the debt the festival had incurred. I felt I had done all I could to them. It was time to move on to other glorious triumphs.

Apparently my dreadful performance at the film festival dinner had made our current governor, Scott Matheson, laugh, too. His assistant called me the next week and asked if I'd come visit the governor. He told me he wanted me to come work for him. He had in mind some job for me that had to do with the arts, as he thought that's where my skills lay. But there was no particular opening in those departments. Then he remembered that I was good with the downtrodden and handicapped, and he settled on asking me to be his assistant for community relations. I would have to give up my newspaper column, but after thirteen years it was just as well. I had just written a column about my little friend Shannon and her jump rope, and her mom called to tell me, "It was even better than the first time you wrote it ten years ago." So it was time to move on anyway.

As it turned out, my job was to meet with all the people the rest of the staff did not wish to see. This included the blind, the deaf, the mentally handicapped, war veterans, and people who believed they were being chased by aliens from a planet far, far away. My problem is that I personally believe anything anyone tells me, and I do my darnedest to make things right, so I found myself checking for interplanetary aliens on the street and asking the governor to help with all sorts of impossible tasks for people who continued to concentrate on larger issues.

When I ventured into the larger issues, I learned that a cat in the form of another staffer would come and bite my ankle, big time. One day the state geologist, who was my pal, came to my office and put his head in his hands. "It's the MX missile project," he said. "The Pentagon wants to install this giant racetrack out in our west desert. Cars with missiles will be going around on it. One missile will be the real thing, the others will be fake, and the Russians won't know which is which."

"You have got to be kidding me. It sounds like little boys playing."

"I know. Here's the thing, though: we don't have the water to make the cement for it and no one seems to be noticing." His face scrunched up. "I've tried to tell the governor this is the stupidest plan ever for this state. I can't even get in to see him. Can you help?"

I went straight to the governor's office, and he beckoned me in. I began to tell him what the state geologist had told me when one of his staff chiefs came in and said they had an urgent matter to deal with, so I should leave.

Later, this same man found me in the hall and said through clenched teeth: "Now you listen to me. I don't care if we cement the whole state over if it means jobs for Utahns. You stay out of this issue!"

"Do you think we have enough water for this brilliant project?"

"I don't care. We are going to get this contract!"

He made sure I was transferred out of the governor's office soon after that.

They don't fire you. They transfer you with a raise so you won't make any trouble. I found this out when I ventured out of my cubicle in the new department and found lots of others in cubicles, all of whom had either blown a whistle or stood up for some principle their boss didn't like. I left after six weeks, raise notwithstanding.

It was right about then that the leaders of the LDS church sent out a position paper against the whole missile project. "We did not travel to this state to be a warlike people," the statement suggested. That was all it took. The MX missile project was dead in Utah, and it never came to pass in any other state either.

Back home, coming up from the laundry room again, I noticed another audition call at the University Theater, this time for the *next* best musical: *Damn Yankees*.

Despite my previous experience, I knew immediately that I should go try out for the part of Lola, the devil's sexy temptress. Of course I could get that role! Sorting socks has a way of blurring reality for me, and once again I hied over to the theater to sign up.

When I auditioned with the song, "A Little Brains, A Little Talent," I felt I had done well. The stage manager came back to pat me on the back. "Terrell. You got a callback."

A callback! That must mean I'm in the running for Lola!

"They want you to come back at four today, to try out for the part of Doris."

"Doris? Who the hell is Doris?"

"She's Sister's friend! You know, the dowdy old neighbor lady in curlers?"

I could not have been more deflated. But I went home and

thought about my place in this world. I guess we have no idea how we appear to other people. I didn't cry, I just went upstairs and changed into a frowsy housedress and orthopedic shoes, put pincurls and a bandana on my head, found a big bag to hit men with, and went back and nailed the part.

I came to love old Doris, especially as I watched the gorgeous dancer they brought in from New York to play Lola. I could never have sung or danced her part, no matter how hard I worked. I finally, cleverly, noticed that when you cannot remember more than two steps in a row, it's a pretty good bet you could not be a Broadway dancer. And it dawned on me at last that singing requires a strong voice that you use over and over, every night. What a revelation!

Never mind. I had the time of my life. The role of the older Joe Hardy was played by Robert Peterson, the baritone who sang "The Impossible Dream" at the Don Quixote Luncheon. For the curtain call each night, we in the cast held hands and sang, "You Gotta Have Heart," and Robert would squeeze my hand every time, letting me know he loved singing at the luncheons where we awarded people for their kindnesses to mentally handicapped kids. It was six weeks of heaven.

On closing night, Mom gave me an ivory heart on a green silk braided chain. With it was a small gold medal, imprinted with the words, "To Terrell, who has more heart than Lola and Doris put together." I think Mom knew how badly I wished to be Lola, and how very Doris I really was, curlers, sensible shoes, and all, and she loved me anyway.

I had even more to say to Michelle, the supervised apartment coordinator who told me to get a life. I wanted to say, Listen, sweet lamb. Before you were born, we women witnessed a lot of change happening around us. First, we were told to get married and have children and stay home and be good moms, and then the feminists came along and said no, no, that isn't really it. You are only one divorce away from poverty, so prepare yourself, get your briefcase, and get out there and have a career. We who loved making raspberry jam and baking cookies with the children felt pretty stupid, watching the younger set move on out and up.

At the time, I interviewed the glamorous feminist Gloria Steinem, and I told her that as a stay-at-home mom, I was a little confused about what was the best life to lead. She laughed and said, "We switched pictures on you in the magazines, didn't we?" I told her yes, and the thing that offended me most was the declaration that it was a waste of time and talent making jam, because it was better in the supermarkets. That's what Betty Freidan said in her book *The Feminine Mystique,* and boy, did *that* take the wind out of our sails, we jam makers, we homemakers. And then, Michelle, get this: just a few years later, Betty Freidan retired and said her very favorite new activity was (wait for it): making jam! Yes! And her best recipe was raspberry! I wanted to poke her with a stick.

So see, Michelle, there's no right answer for me, or for you, either. I promise you that I have a life. And during that life, I have seen sadness, boredom, and frustration in young stay-at-home mothers, but I have to tell you, I haven't seen such joyous looks on the faces of earnest young women carrying those briefcases and wearing pin-striped suits, either. In fact, they look just as tired as full-time homemakers. So what the hell, Michelle? We all have a life, we try to get the best life we can, we live many lives in our lifetime. And we're just trying to take care of ourselves, and each other, as well and as lovingly as we can.

13

Family Struggling Please Help

Weight gain occurs a lot in the mentally disabled population as it grows older, and the problem is a real health issue. Diabetes is always right on the horizon. Irene had gained seventy pounds in two years.

So when we brought her to family dinners, each family member in turn would subtly bring up all the joys of being a bit more in shape. "Boy, Irene, it looks to me like you're on the road to getting thinner. Is that right?"

"I am?"

"Yes! Imagine how gorgeous you'll be when you're thin!"

"And what happens then?"

"Well, Irene, um, let's see. I know! You can wear a bikini!"

"And . . . what happens when I wear a bikini?

"All the boys will whistle at you!"

"And what happens when they whistle at me?"

"Maybe you can go on a date!"

"And what happens when I go on a date?"

"Um . . . well, you go out and have fun and have dinner and go the movies!"

"Like I do now? I could have nachos and cheese at the movie? Like I do now?"

"Um, sure." By now the family member's eyes have glazed over, realizing she is so far ahead of us all on the subject that we have no arguments left. She would wait for a few seconds and then ask, "What's for dessert?"

Besides, she was refusing to go to work at the sheltered workshop. Her staff was going through hell, begging her, bribing her, but she had dug her heels in. She wanted to stay home and snack all day and watch TV.

My uncle Bob had been calling and nagging me about Irene and the quality of her life. I knew he loved her, but he was like so many of my friends who just didn't have the tools to cope with her. Now and then he'd invite her to lunch and give her a dollar or two, but mostly their relationship was long distance and through me.

He kept quizzing me, like some armchair quarterback, adding to my sense of total responsibility.

"Why is she so far away out there in West Valley City in that apartment?"

"Because that's where the program is, Bob. It's really close to her sheltered workshop."

"Why did she have that cut on her forehead last week when she came here to lunch?"

"She had a dust-up with the girl who lives upstairs. They have really hated each other for years."

"Well, move her!"

"Bob, I can't just move her! She's in a system!"

"Why?"

I wanted to scream. I told Bob I had to go, hung up, and yelled to the gods, "Help! I need some direction here!"

Sometimes you have to yell at them. And then wait.

Irene's social worker, Susan, called me and said, "Guess what. It turns out other parents and siblings are frustrated with their kids' programs too, and now there's a new option for you, where you get to do the hiring and firing of staff if you can find a home for the special-needs person. Want to find her her own place and run her program? It's called SAM, the self-administered model. People in the government are crazy about it because it puts a lot of the work about hiring and firing on you, not them. I guess they're tired of trying to find caretakers for these kids. Do you blame them?"

No. I could not blame them.

The idea of being able to choose Irene's companions sounded good to me.

"Do you think I could?"

"What are you talking about? You helped *design* the whole group home program."

"Yes, but, listen: maybe my judgment is way off. Do you think I'm a codependent person?" Susan had listened to my complaints about Irene's program for two years.

"Hell, yes. So am I. So what? It's our karma to make things better. You have Irene, I have forty other Irenes I work with all day, every day. Terrell, go for it! Find a place and get Irene's program the way you want it. Please yourself. The state can pay a good portion of the staffing money. It saves the state money because you would provide the home. The fiscal agent takes care of all the withholding taxes, so you're not going to be drowned in paperwork. Just consider switching to this model."

I told her to send me the application papers.

Then I thought, what the hell have I done? Should I rent a home? How long could the trust afford that?

Uncle Bob Shows His True Colors

Uncle Bob, Mom's little brother, scared Bammy every day of his life with his dangerous antics with go-carts and pranks on the trolley tracks with his buddies. Bammy was just grateful he had never been seriously hurt. He was tall, handsome, and very attractive to women. Irene and I were his only living relatives. He had watched from the sidelines as our family went through the process of rearing Irene, and now he was badgering me about her.

But very soon after I decided to make my own way with Irene's living arrangements, Uncle Bob called me up and invited me to lunch. He was now eighty-six, his thick hair was now white, and the ladies at his assisted-living facility were stopping by the table to invite him for cocktails.

After lunch, he sat back. I was waiting for another quiz on how I might improve Irene's life. Instead he said, "Why don't we buy Irene a house?"

"Bob, I don't think Mom and Dad left enough money for all that. Well, I could buy a small house, but then the cost of maintenance would run the trust out in a few years."

"But I would buy the house."

"Good Lord, Bob, with what?"

"Turns out I've made a few bucks with that money Bam left me. I got really interested in investing it, and I think I have enough to buy her a little house, maybe a duplex. Why don't we look in the Avenues so she'd be close to you?"

"Bobby. I am stunned."

"Well, hell, Tiger, I can't take it with me. Why not? I think this is just what she needs. Face it: she doesn't want to be with kids like her. She hits them. Why not do her and them a favor? Let's go for it." With that, he picked up his phone and called his favorite realtor.

When I told the people at the supervised apartment project, they were really upset. "Well," said one manager, a really fine person who runs a good program, "I'll tell you who's losing out here. It's Irene. She will be protected and babied and waited on, the way you want her to be. It doesn't serve her well."

This went straight to my neurotic little heart, and I spent many more sleepless nights, fighting with myself, tossing and turning, over what was best for Irene. Finally Paul sat up and bed and said, "Listen. It's time you get to please yourself in this area. I'm interested in your getting some sleep, you know? This will in turn let me get *my* sleep, and we can go forward with our lives. Terrell, put a program together that works for you as well as Irene. What does a good program look like to you?"

As I began to talk, the talk turned into a whine and then a sob. "I want her clean and busy and happy and *healthy*—she's almost a hundred pounds overweight because of the candy machine—and participating in the life of the community in a way that suits *her,* not me, and not her staff."

"Well, now, that shouldn't be too hard to achieve, do you think? You hire good staff, you pay them well, so well they don't leave. You give them a set of operating instructions. You know what she likes, you know what triggers her tantrums. You tell them. Then you hire a cleaning woman. You get a good psychiatric professional who knows the latest in medications to help even Irene out. For God's sake, Terrell. Just please *yourself.* Be in charge. Don't try to please anyone else. Don't even try to please Irene for right now. Find the house, follow your instincts. Just get out there and do it. You have some of the resources, and the state has given you the power with their new program. Stop taking this out of your own hide. Go to sleep now, and in the morning get on with it."

"Easy for you to say. You're not living this."

"Oh yeah? It's two in the morning. Believe me, baby, I'm living this."

We found a charming little house in the Avenues, a duplex on two floors, very near the J Street home where Irene and I had grown up, the street I've always felt held magic because we had so much fun there in the 1950s. Some of our old neighbors were still living in their homes. When I went to see them, they were delighted to see us both again. We speculated about getting a game of kick the can going on a summer evening, even though our hair was graying.

Irene's duplex had a garden that needed a lot of work, but that made it kind of fun, I thought. I loved the idea of her having her own private home. I would run my own version of the least restrictive alternative. She could be out and about in her neighborhood! Her neighbors would come to love her, I just knew it.

First, her health program. Having gained so much weight in the supervised-apartment program, Irene had developed diabetes and high blood pressure. In order to bring her blood pressure down, she had to walk a lot. Remembering Glenn Latham's great teaching about behavior modification, I thought of what motivated Irene, and the answer was right under my nose: going to visit her heroes, the firemen, and getting money.

The fire station was only six blocks from Irene's house. I went to see the firemen and explained my goals for Irene. I asked them, if I gave them an envelope full of one-dollar bills, would they give Irene a high five and hand her a dollar every time she came to visit? They could send her home again with her dollar, and I didn't think she'd bother them too much. They said they'd be happy to help.

Then I went to LDS Hospital, where they have a gift shop. I asked the ladies who worked there if they would consider a layaway program for trinkets Irene wanted. I explained about her program of visiting the firemen and receiving a dollar and a high five from them. Could she walk to the hospital, only three blocks from her house, and put some money down on some item she wanted to buy, and when she had paid in full, take her treasure home? The gift shop ladies agreed.

Some nurses nearby overheard me. "Wait a minute," they said, "You mean you're giving your sister a dollar to go walk over to those adorable firemen? Could *we* get on that program?"

Next: hiring the companion.

One of her helpers at her old program, Janie, a beautiful young woman, asked me to hire her as Irene's companion. After all, she knew her well and was already trained to work with Irene. Besides, Irene loved her. She was willing to follow my new rules for a clean house and dry laundry. Besides, she needed a place to live while she figured out her future. "But Janie," I said, "you are drop-dead gorgeous. You'll be dating or getting married before we know it."

"I have no boyfriend," she replied. "None."

Well, it was perfect. Everything was going to be all right.

WHAT HAPPENED NEXT was that Janie announced she was pregnant. She had been having a fight with her boyfriend when she applied for the job with Irene. Now she was going to marry him and have the baby, but could they stay anyway? They needed a place to live.

I asked Irene about it, and she said that would be a good thing because she loved babies. Irene, dressed to the nines, was in Janie's wedding as the guest book lady.

Meanwhile, Irene longed for a hot tub in her backyard. Once again, Uncle Bob came to the rescue. "Why not?" he asked. "Life is short. Get a hot tub."

So we built one, and that's when we got to know Irene's neighbors, the Hansons. The Hansons have a perfect view right down into Irene's backyard. They had been very accepting and welcoming when we first moved Irene in, and I explained about Irene and the living arrangement. They were especially pleased with the beautiful garden we put in. All seemed to be going well. Then one day Mary Hanson came to see me as I was getting into the car in Irene's driveway.

"We are very concerned about Irene and that hot tub," she said.

"Why is that?"

"She gets in there with her doll. Then if she sees Bill or me, she calls to us and starts a conversation. Sometimes she is talking about her doll being a naughty girl and then she holds the doll under the water for a long time. Do you think she'd do that to Janie's baby?"

I laughed aloud. They had no idea about Irene. But on the way home, I began to fret that maybe this was what Irene was thinking, as she could be very jealous of the baby as Janie took care of it.

Paul found me tossing and turning in the night again. "Now what?" he said.

"Oh, nothing. Just program problems."

"It never ends, does it?"

"Nope. But I'm happier having her closer." I reminded myself to tell Janie of the Hansons' concern and warn her.

When I did tell Janie, she laughed too. "Never gonna happen," she said. "Irene would never in the world do that, nor would I ever have my baby in a hot tub. Relax!'

On the one hand, I fretted about neighbors complaining about every little thing. On the other hand, I was grateful that they would keep an extra eye out for me.

Over the years, the Hansons have been Irene's best friends and great neighbors. Once Irene had to have oral surgery and I brought her home very sedated because she had been put under anesthesia. It was all I could do to get her in the house. Mary, seeing us out her window, came running and put one of Irene's arms over her shoulder to help me. "Let me help you get Irene to bed. I love this lady."

When Janie's baby Molly was born, Irene carried her around, helped feed her, and reveled in the whole scene of surrogate motherhood. I peeked in the kitchen window once and found Irene feeding the baby in her high chair, talking to the baby as if she were her doll. Janie and her little family lived with Irene for almost three years, until the next baby was due and we all simply ran out of room.

We then found Kay, Irene's head staff member and house manager, and three other wonderful young women, to make up Irene's staff. All was progressing nicely. Kay, who had worked in other group home programs, knew how important Irene's independence was to her. She bought Irene a bus pass to use on her way to work at an incense factory and back. Irene was easily trained to make a bus transfer and get to her job, where her job coach was waiting. She loved the bus pass that hung around her neck.

It's just that sometimes, as we all do, she liked to take a left turn and not get on the second bus at all. After all, there were all those shops at the mall.

To All Employees of ZCMI Mall:

The person in this picture is my sister, Irene Harris. She has a mental disability and cannot read or write. She takes the bus to work in an incense factory three days a week. She loves the independence and the mall. But yesterday apparently she got hold of her checkbook, which must have two signatures, and went up to the Time Shop guys, and bought a $200 watch, asking the clerk to fill in the right amount. Then she went downstairs and signed up for her own cell phone by showing her ID card to the salesman at the cell phone kiosk. After she bought a purse from you guys at Deseret Bookstore, she went to Bruce down at the Beauty Spa and ordered a hair cut.

When Bruce finished, she said, "Oh, I don't have any money," and left. She had used up all her checks and just smiled at Bruce. I have gone round and returned the phone and the watch and thanks for tearing up the checks, and I've paid Bruce, who said he didn't need to be paid because he just loved being with Irene, but this is to ask you please not to let her do this again.

We try to watch and supervise her, but she also treasures her independence, and we try not to restrict her more than is absolutely necessary. My phone number is listed below, along with her helpers who work for me, and please call us if she is out on a grand shopping spree again.

Thanks for any help you can give us in this matter. And thanks for loving and supporting Irene.

Terrell Dougan

P.S. I did let her keep the purse.

Soon afterward, I bought Irene a cell phone. You'd think a cell phone would help, but think again. Now that she has one, here's how it goes.

"Irene, hi! We've been looking for you! Where are you?"

"I'm right here!" she says happily.

"Yes, but where is here?"

"Right here!" She cannot believe we can't tell where that is.

"Honey, what's around you? Do you see a sign?"

"Yes!"

"Yes, good. Now what is on that sign?"

"It's the sign for the bus stop!"

"Is someone standing by you?"

"Yes! Want to talk to him?"

"Yes. Put him on."

She does. "Hello."

"Hi. I'm her sister. Can you tell me where you are?"

And if he can, then I can take it from there.

What we soon learned was that she became very adept at calling any phone number she saw on any poster, just to chat.

The Incident of the Lost Dog

Lady Who Lost Dog: Hello?

Irene: Hi! This is Irene! Who's this?

LWLD: Have you found my dog?

Irene: I saw his picture on a poster here! He's a cute dog.

LWLD: Oh, thank God. Where are you?

Irene: I'm right here!

LWLD: Is it by the bus stop on Tenth Ave? That poster?

Irene: Yes! I'm here!

LWLD: Do you see my dog right there?

Irene (looking at poster): Yes! I see him right here! He's cute!

LWLD: Keep him right there! I'm on my way! Don't leave there, okay?

Irene: Okay.

The lady and her husband arrived at the bus stop in their car. Irene pointed to the poster and smiled. Then the lady asked where the dog was, and of course Irene pointed to the poster. Then the lady demanded to know where Irene lived, and since it was only two blocks away, she took them there. They came up her stairs and demanded to know where the dog was being kept. Kay said they were not harboring any lost dog. These poor folks took a complete tour of the duplex and the backyard, feeling sure Irene wanted some reward money or something. When it was finally clear to them that Irene just liked to dial numbers on posters and chat, they asked, "Well, what sort of fool would give someone like that a cell phone?"

Kay finally arranged with the cell phone company for Irene

to receive calls on that phone but not make them. At least now we know how to find her. ("Honey, where are you?" "I'm right here!")

Irene knows exactly where she is. *We* are the ones who have a problem.

I continued to believe everything would be all right. I told myself so every day.

One day Irene and I were downtown and crossing Main Street. When we were halfway across Irene dropped her purse, and the light changed, so Irene ran to safety across the street, looking back anxiously at her purse on the street. She was sure the cars would run over her purse, with her money and her cell phone in it. She began to scream. A homeless woman was standing nearby, holding up a sign that said: "Family Struggling Please Help."

Still screaming, Irene found a fire hydrant, where she leaned over and began banging her head on it. Everyone on the street was staring, dumbfounded. I looked at the woman and said, "Can I borrow your sign?"

She started to laugh, and then a homeless man with dreadlocks and a big backpack came loping across the street. He grabbed Irene's purse, ran straight to Irene, and held it out to her. "Here! Lady! Here's your purse! Stop bangin' your head!"

She stopped, took her purse, wiped her tears, and thanked him. I gave them some money by way of thanks, as well.

We went home, and I kept thinking I could not cope anymore and that maybe I had made a horrid mistake in taking charge of her program. At the time I was too frazzled to realize all the color Irene adds to my days.

I am not a religious person. But that night, just like my father before me, I got down on my knees and asked for the Lord's help.

I was crying, and I felt totally alone and scared that I was not up to this job.

I asked for strength and guidance. I told him/her that I was turning everything over to the higher power, and into its hands I commended my spirit. When I stood up, I remembered the last time I really prayed, instead of playfully shouting to my various gods in the universe. I had been twelve years old and we were driving away to a new house. I was looking back at my childhood home and my willow tree at 518 J Street, and asking to be allowed to go back there. I remember promising God I would do anything to get back there. And it occurred to me that when I was twelve, I was asking for my childhood home back. Now I was just asking for strength and guidance. Maybe that's what a person should pray for, I thought. I mean, God isn't Santa Claus.

I felt better, just asking for help, and the next morning I went to the phone book and called the Mormons, some of them the very same people we went to church with as children in our neighborhood. I told a woman on the other end of the line that Irene was going to be a new member of the ward, which is like a neighborhood parish.

She said, "Well, I just know Bishop Coles will be thrilled to have her."

"Coles? You don't mean Bob Coles?" I had dated this lovely man years ago in junior high school. He was always wonderful with Irene when he came to my house.

"Yes, Bob Coles. I'll have him visit Irene this week."

I hung up the phone and burst into tears. Somehow God heard something and was right there. The next Sunday, Irene and I went to Relief Society together.

The Relief Society of the Church of Jesus Christ of Latter-day

Saints, the Mormons, was formed back in 1842 by church founder Joseph Smith, who knew how powerful women were in healing and helping each other. It is an organization of women for women. If you are sick, they'll bring food and tend your children. If you are new in the neighborhood, they're on your doorstep with an elegant Bundt cake or hot homemade bread, offering themselves at your service. They were delighted to have Irene as a member. I told them I couldn't come much myself, and they said, "Oh, that's fine. Just have her helper drop her off to us, and we'll take care of the rest."

I had a writer friend in New York whose husband was an out-of-work actor. They were almost living hand-to-mouth. We were on the phone, and I said, "Gotta go. I'm taking Irene to Relief Society for her first time."

"What's a Relief Society?" asked my friend.

I explained it to her.

"I want one! I want a Relief Society," she whimpered.

Of course these women live all through the neighborhood. When Irene goes for walks, I know they are watching out for her through their windows, and I know she is safe. Let me tell you: if your family has troubles, if there is flood, earthquake, or famine, I highly recommend living among the Mormons. They are the most organized, prepared, kind, and generous people I know. Even though I don't go to church anymore, I think of them as my people. While I don't subscribe to the theologies in their faith, and I get frustrated with their suppression of academics who ask hard questions, I adore their culture of community and caring. And I'll hold up their homemade ice cream against any in the world. When a voter these days asks, "What can you do with the Mormons?" My answer is simple: you can count on them.

The Pink Prescription

I took one more step toward making a comfortable home for Irene. It sounds very farfetched and silly, but I had Irene's bedroom painted Baker-Miller pink. In 1979, two officers at a naval prison facility in Seattle read the work of psychologists who found that a certain shade of pink had a positive effect on prisoners who were extremely violent. Officers Baker and Miller, at their wits' end with these violent guys, got the paint color formula (very close to Benjamin Moore number 1328), matched it, and painted their receiving room this color. Ignoring the laughing remarks of their fellow officers about their sexual orientation, they put their violent prisoners in this pink holding cell for fifteen minutes. To their amazement, the prisoners quieted right down. They sent the results to the psychologists, who then proceeded to test it in other prisons, and now we have the color Baker-Miller pink, which is still in use today at many facilities to bring a little peace and tranquility to those who feel frantic and aggressive.

I'm not sure the Baker-Miller pink really worked. But it made me feel good about trying every avenue toward Irene's improved peace of mind and calmer behavior.

There was still the problem of the children in the neighborhood. I didn't want her to be the object of ridicule, as she was when she lived with Dana in a different neighborhood. Here, no one had teased Irene or been cruel to her, but the children were a little afraid of her, really. When she would call to them and wave from her front porch, they often ducked inside or around to their backyards. I had no idea how to fix that. I had to hand that one over to the higher powers, as well.

One hot summer day Irene called to say, "I'm having a lemonade stand. Wanna come?"

"Of course," I said.

"I invited my firemen, too."

"Honey," I said, "the firemen have to watch out for fires. I don't think they'll be able to come."

"Well, I invited 'em."

An hour went by, and I decided to go visit her. I was afraid maybe the neighborhood kids would laugh at a grown lady selling lemonade, and I might be her only customer. So when I rounded the corner to her front lawn, my jaw fell open.

Two fire engines were parked in front of her house, and her front lawn was lousy with firemen, drinking lemonade. The neighborhood kids were climbing around the fire trucks, in awe of this special lady with her special friends.

The firemen had launched her socially for all time. These heroes show up in the most amazing places.

14

Adventures in Community Life

To Janet James, Owner, The Incense Factory

From: Terrell Dougan, Irene Harris's sister

Dear Janet:

I want to thank you again for giving Irene the chance to work at your factory, and I hope you'll let me explain about our current predicament. Irene loves garage sales, especially her own. Every Saturday morning in good weather she puts her card table up and displays a poster saying everything is one dollar.

Then she gets all the little stuffed animals she bought at All-A-Dollar over the year and puts them out to sell, along with other bits of costume jewelry and coloring books, etc. She has no idea about how much her initial inventory cost. She just wants money in her pocket. So apparently this summer her enterprise made her think of bigger and better things. She wanted to expand her inventory but had no real budget to do it.

So she began to think of your hundreds of boxes of precious oils to scent the incense. Irene began to take a few home in her purse each day after work. When I saw her selling them, I assumed either you had given them to her or she had bought them with the few dollars she's allowed to carry in her wallet. I had no idea the oils cost $10 a vial and you personally watched her filch some from each box!

To show you what an entrepreneur she is, she was selling $10 vials of oil for $1. We are extremely embarrassed that she chose to expand her inventory in this fashion, and I am enclosing a check for the ten vials she has stolen. If you find more gone, please let me know. I have asked her companions to frisk her every day when she comes home, and I certainly agree with you that she cannot be allowed to bring big purses to the factory! I am floored that you haven't fired her already, and am grateful you'll give her one more chance. I'm not sure she deserves it, and at the same time, I'm not sure she really understood that she was stealing. We have discussed the matter with her, and she says she understands that she cannot take the vials anymore. I hope this is true.

But my advice is, keep frisking on your end, and we will too. Among the new skills she is learning, such as bus transfers, I had no idea she would include having sticky fingers as a main goal.

Sincerely,

Terrell Dougan

Irene has had many different jobs over the years. Once, she cleaned toilets at Sutherland Lumber and made more than she's ever made before or since. During that time, she was strolling around with as much as $70 in her pocket: all money she had earned and had a right to spend as she chose. It was, after all, her money. She was so excited the day she cashed her first paycheck with Sutherland for

$72. She invited me to lunch and chose the Red Rock Brewery, a place I had taken her the week before. That week, she had started hitting herself and yelling, "I don't like it here!" So we left.

But now, she pointed at it and said, "Let's go here."

"You wouldn't go here last week."

"I changed my mind. I want to take you to lunch here. My treat."

We went in and she said to the head waiter, "Two, please." When we sat down she said, "You bring me the check at the end, please?"

During that lunch I felt as if I had a completely delightful sister. We talked and laughed over a delicious lunch. When the waiter brought the check, she pulled out her wallet and paid, somehow knowing that she'd still have a lot left over.

I was floored. I had found the secret to Irene's sadness and bad behavior: she felt powerless without money in her pocket! If she had money, and quite a bit of it, she became amenable. I felt like Oliver Sacks discovering the dopamine component in patients with Alzheimer's.

So the next week, as an experiment, I gave her $40, just for walking-around money, to see what would happen with her behavior. She invited one of her companions to go out to lunch, her treat.

When the bill came, she handed it to the companion.

"I thought you were buying today," said the companion.

"No! No!" she yelled, and bit her knuckle. "It's my money! I have to have my money!"

Fortunately, the companion had money that day, and rather than cause more of a scene, she paid.

It has been that way ever since, no matter how much she has in her wallet. She wants to feel powerful and treat you, but in the end, she refuses to pay.

Actually, I know several men and women just like that, don't you?

But I really miss the woman I met that day at Red Rock. She has never returned, and I don't know where she went or how to bring her back.

Most of the time Irene's money would go to baby dolls and doll clothing. When she quit the Sutherland job because it was a forty-five-minute drive from her home and the bus route was too confusing for her, her income went down considerably, but her desires and spending habits didn't. I had all the expenses I could handle, so her walking-around money had to go way down.

> To: Walt at the Eighth Avenue Market
>
> From: Terrell Dougan, sister of your friend Irene
>
> I am so very sorry, Walt, to hear of Irene's visit to you yesterday. I had no idea she was headed your way; she told us she was going to the public library. When I heard that she filled a small grocery cart to the top with candy bars and then tried to buy it from you with two dollars, you must have been furious. I am sorry you had to put all the candy back yourself. Irene cannot read or write and needs to be told, if she comes in again, that she can buy chewing gum, diet Coke, or coloring books, but no candy. I am so sorry, again, to place you in this position. We are trying to give Irene the least restrictive life she can lead, but she's obviously playing us for complete suckers. We'll get a better handle on this community living soon. You were a saint to be so kind to her.

You must have talked to her and understood about her limitations.

Thank you, and your employees, for your many kindnesses to Irene.

Her sister, Terrell

What Is Normal?

In the field of mental disabilities, the word "normalization" creeps into the vocabulary fairly often. It means two things: one, you try to have the person with the disability act as normally as possible; and two, you try to get the community used to having this person around. This is called normalizing the community. It means making sure those citizens with special needs have the chance and the right to be out and about in the community, instead of segregated and protected in a place far away. Eventually, the theory goes, our "normal" citizens will realize that these citizens do and will live among us and they'd better get used to it.

Here's an example of normalizing: My friend Carolyn's daughter Annette, a young woman with Down syndrome, was in front of me in the grocery store. I had watched her grow up and now she was in a group home. She and the other women from the group home were out getting their groceries, all together. They were very slow at putting each item from the cart onto the conveyor belt. People in the line behind us were getting impatient and whispering to each other. The group home staff member stepped out of line and looked back at them and said, "This is your tax dollars at work, folks!" And he gave them a beaming smile.

People laughed and smiled back. The tension was over. He

had normalized the community in a small way, in just a moment. We in the volunteer force and we siblings have laughed about normalizing the country club, normalizing the legislature, you name it.

And when you really look at behaviors, I mean maybe those of your friends, don't you have to ask yourself what the hell "normal" is?

Professionals tell us it is not normal for Irene to stuff herself with candy. One of my best, high-IQ friends stuffs herself with candy daily.

Oh, but it's not normal to carry those dolls around! Yet one of the most intelligent women I know has a magnificent doll collection, and is often seen carrying her dolls. She has many more dolls than Irene does. The only difference is, this woman does not ask you to *talk* to her dolls.

So we're constantly thinking how to get Irene to appear "normal" in as many ways as possible. The rule on dolls is that of course she can collect them, but not take them with her and make people talk to them.

Fashion: Let's Be Appropriate

In addition to working on behaviors, we work on appearance.

I have a theory that some special-needs people actually like having special needs. It gets them a lot more care, kindness, and attention than they would otherwise get. Irene is walking proof. She loves Mickey Mouse knee socks, worn with shorts, no matter what the weather. The moment my back was turned, all through our times together, Irene would get into this outfit.

Years ago, a study was done on this very topic. The people running the study offered to dress a group of special-needs young adults in the latest fashions. They offered wigs. They offered makeup. They even offered glasses with clear glass in them, just to make these kids look smarter. Then they took their pictures, placed the pictures in an album along with pictures of regular people, and asked a large sampling of folks to identify the special-needs kids. Well, no one could, really. This then proved their point—that appearance really helps in the self-esteem department! Another master's thesis was finished. The special-needs subjects thanked them, cheered for them, and sent them on their way.

But here's the rub: the minute the people departed, all these subjects who had been fussed with and dressed differently went right back to their high dutch boy bangs and little stylistic touches, like huge rings of keys on their belts and fuzzy animal purses. They liked themselves that way. So much for helping them out. They knew who they were. Once again, we're the ones who have the problem.

It's certainly ongoing in our lives. When Irene and I attended a funeral just last week, she showed up in her driveway in a summer dress (it was thirty degrees outside) and her socks were nylons that came up midcalf. I said, "Oh, no. Oh no, no, no," and got out of the car to make her change her socks.

Marriott and Paul were with me. "Mom," said Mare, "it's okay! Let it go! We're going to be late anyway, and Irene looks fine."

"Fine? You think she looks fine? She can't go like this."

Irene, used to my fashion fits, climbed into the car and waited to see what would happen next. I ran into her house, searched through her sock drawers for something other than Mickey

Mouse socks, and came up empty-handed. I grabbed a warm coat and raced out.

"Mom!" Mare said. "It's fine. Let it go."

So we went to the funeral, Irene happy and me fuming. The fact that no one noticed was not the point. The point was that Mother was haunting me with every fiber of her being. "You make sure Irene looks presentable. Every day!"

I invited Irene to a Valentine's Day ladies' luncheon recently. As people began to arrive, I got a phone call from Kay, her chief companion. "I've tried everything to get her into the black velvet pants and top with the red heart necklace. She will have none of it. We fought for two hours. She is in Levis and an old red sweater with a hood. I'm sorry, I've done everything I could."

When she arrived, I took her aside and said, "I have half a mind to send you home until you can come back in a nice party outfit! Why do you keep doing this to me?"

She said, "You have a Valentine present for me?"

I was close to sending her back home when another guest arrived. To my amazement, the guest was also wearing very baggy jeans.

Irene and I welcomed her and led her into my house. When the guest's back was turned, Irene caught my eye and put both her hands over her mouth, stifling laughter, her eyes twinkling.

"Oh, Irene," I said, "I'm sorry. See how wrong I am. You should wear what you like. Will you forgive me?"

"I'give ya. I can have that Valentine present now?"

"Sure. Honey, what's wrong with me, do you think?"

She put her arm around me. "Your brain isn't awake yet."

I thought of the magnet Irene has on her refrigerator:

NORMAL PEOPLE WORRY ME.

15

Confessions of a Codependent

When Michelle yelled at me that I was a raging codependent, I decided to find out exactly what that condition is, and researched it. Here's what I've come up with so far.

Codependency means you're hooked on having someone depend on you. In other words, you need desperately to be needed. You hover around people, hoping to be helpful. In other words, you are pathetic.

The condition starts in childhood, they say, when you see extreme stress in your family and you begin to think it falls to you to fix it. You try and try to make the problems go away, and they just don't go away.

Some romantic twit has written a song that tells you to make someone happy, and then you will be happy, too.

I've spent most of my life trying to make just one someone happy, and it has made me a slightly crazed woman with a lot of headaches. I know it's nice to try to accommodate other people's needs, but some of us take it way over the top. I've devised my own test for this condition.

How to Tell if You're Codependent

1. Do you lie awake at night, furious at your sister's helper who wouldn't let her have a third ice-cream cone, even though you know that she has diabetes?

2. Can you go to a family party and not ask if they'll please invite your special-needs sibling? And when they do (with a sigh), are you surprised to find that the sibling didn't want to go anyway?

3. Can you buy yourself a purse without buying your sister a purse, too? How about a wristwatch? Can you get a manicure without ordering one for your sister, too?

4. You are the speaker at a luncheon. You get a phone call ten minutes before you're on, and the news is that your sister has wet her pants at the sheltered workshop. No one else is available to go pick your sister up or to bring her dry clothes. Do you:

   a. Leave the luncheon with apologies and go pick her up?

   b. Call the workshop and tell them that you bet she really didn't wet her pants? She has just claimed to have wet her pants because she's bored and wants to go home. You bet that somehow she intuits that you're doing something fancy and she wants to make sure you don't do it. Hang in there: staff will be along in two hours to pick her up.

In the last case, I want you to know that I chose answer b. I was also right about her pants.

Because of past sadness about neighbor children making fun of Irene, I am nuts on that issue too. Children who tease other children, or bully them, bring out the psychopath in me. I myself was bullied by Mean Merrill Hall, who would push me down and wash my face with snow, and I have never gotten over it. When my daughter Marriott was in third grade, a boy who sat behind her, Grant, had a little crush on her, and he did what most boys do in third grade when they get a crush on a girl: he terrorized her. He stuck pins in her, pulled her pigtails, and pummeled her with snowballs on the way home from school. One day she called me from a friend's house, imprisoned in there. Grant was waiting outside with his buddies, snowballs in hand. Marriott asked if I could come pick her up. I did. The boys saw me coming and scattered.

However (and this is why I need so much help on so many levels): the next day, after school, I drove near Grant's house and waited for him to show up. I jumped out of my car, grabbed him, and shoved him against a tree, pinning his arms. "Are you Grant?"

He looked stunned. "Yes."

"Well, Grant, I am Marriott's mother. I want to tell you right now that if you so much as get *near* her again, in school, out of school, wherever, I will come and I will find you, and you will not like what happens next. I will know if you ever touch Mare again. See, Grant, I really, really hate bullies. And you are a bully. I have people watching you. Is there anything about this conversation you don't understand?"

He shook his head, his eyes wide with alarm. I let him go then. I told Mare about it at dinner. "Oh, Mom!" she cried, embarrassed.

"Never you mind, Mare. He will not bother you again."

The next day at school, Grant did actually speak to Mare, quietly and politely. "Mare? Your mom—"

"Yes. My mom." She shook her head.

Grant grinned. "She's so *cool!*"

Years later he came to a party at our house. He stood in my doorway, all six-feet-four of him, looking down at me. He could have snapped me like a twig. "Mrs. Dougan? I'm Grant." Then he laughed and hugged me.

I am fortunate that so many people in my life have forgiven me for marching into untold hells for what I consider a heavenly cause, like Don Quixote.

"Professionals" tell me that I enable my sister to be dependent and needy. They're probably correct. But in my defense, I also try to empower her to lead a more satisfying life. There's a huge difference here, in my mind. You can't completely force a brain-damaged person into self-sufficiency, I don't care how many courses you've taken on the subject. Try living it every day, and you'll see.

Oddly enough, through watching me care for Irene in my over-the-top way, my daughters feel it is their responsibility, too. If I am hit by a truck, they will both be right there to watch out for her, and hire good companions, and be in charge of her program. When I gently broached the subject of what will happen if Irene outlives me, my whole family chimed in: "We'll be here! We'll take care of her! What were you thinking?" They were horrified that I would not consider them as my backups. "In a flood," Paul said, "who do you think is going to go get Irene? Her social worker? Of course we'll be there!"

And through years of expensive therapy, I learned (duh): I have a right to make myself happy, too. And if that means insisting on a clean environment for my sister by hiring a cleaning professional, so be it. The "experts" can shake their heads and say Irene should do it all herself. I have come to believe they're just wishing they could have a cleaning lady, too, and I stand my ground.

There's another problem with being so extra kind to others. We Who Care Too Much absolutely attract those who crave extra care. I swear they can sense us from miles away. Just like heat-seeking missiles, the needy find the need-to-be-needed, and we go into our dance.

The good news about this strange habit enjoyed by so many of us is this: we really do make the world a nicer place. One professional says, "Could it be that people who struggle with that catchall word 'codependency' are really just extra-nice people?"

The bad news is, it tends to make *us* sick. So in an effort to get over my hypertension, sore shoulders, and headaches, I am working on myself all the time. This does not mean I wouldn't rush to help someone who fell down. It just means I don't go around *looking* for people who fell down. There's a difference. I think I really used to do this. It just made my day to help someone.

I found a lovely book for the likes of us. It's called *I Don't Have to Make Everything All Better,* by Gary and Joy Lundberg. My favorite suggestion they have for us is this: when someone comes to tell you the problem, hoping you'll jump in and fix it for them, you say, "My goodness, that really is a problem. What are you going to do?" Their point is, this empowers the person rather than weakens them. Another book, *How to Talk So Kids Will Listen and Listen So Kids Will Talk*, by Adele Faber and Elaine Mazlish, was given to me by my daughter Marriott, now a mother herself, who gently pointed out to me that she did not need me to tell her what to do in every single situation. Her big sister Kate thanked her profusely for giving me the book, but still asks: "What happened? Did you throw it away?"

Here's the lesson I need to learn from these books: when people tell me their problems, they aren't really hoping I'll fix them. They just want me to listen, to get it, and not solve it for them! What a concept! I'm in the autumn of my life, and no one ever pointed this out to me before.

As to my sister, I know she can't really fix a lot of her problems, and wants me to solve them for her, but every day I work toward referring these problems back to her ("What are you going to do about it?") or to her staff. Then I turn back to *my* life.

My sister is a walking ball of needs ("Can we go get a Slurpee? Can you change my quarters for me? Can you come take me for a ride? My lightbulb needs changing. My lamp is broken. My ear hurts. I have a hangnail. My knees hurt"). I make a mental note to refer some of these things to staff, and tell her we'll get them handled one way or another.

But sometimes Irene wants her needs attended to right away. Just last week, around noon one day, I called to check on her.

"Hi, Irene, how's it going?"

"I'm mad. I'm all alone, and I'm hungry!" (She begins to cry pitifully.)

"Where's Kay?"

"Gone! She left me!"

"Did she come this morning? Did you get breakfast?"

"No! No one! Nothing! I'm here all alone!" (Sobbing now.)

My head starts to ache, anger stirs my adrenaline; I hang up and try to get Kay on the line, but she's not answering her cell phone. I'm already thinking of how fast I can get an ad in the paper for a new helper, because surely Kay is going to be fired. I make a sandwich and head up to Irene's house, where I see Kay just pulling in.

"Where have you been?" I ask her.

"Getting our lunch at the grocery store," she answers.

"But you never came this morning."

"What are you talking about? I came, helped her fix breakfast, and then told her we were going to buy a new telephone, because hers was broken. She got mad at me for some reason, and threw the phone at me, just missing my head. So I left, and have been getting the new phone and our lunch."

I was holding the lunch I'd made Irene and looking pretty stupid. We both went inside to confront Irene. "You lied to me, Irene," I said to her.

"Yeah, I got breakfast already. Is that my lunch?" she said, looking at the sack I was holding and also the sack Kay was holding.

Two lunches. Exactly what she was aiming for, once I'd called her. Believe me, she is no dummy. (No, she did not get both lunches. I ate the one I made for her. And then the one I made for me.) At times like these, she manipulates all of us any which way she wants. Do you suppose she has *War and Peace* stashed under her bed, and this is all a big show for more care and attention? How can she keep outsmarting me?

One thing I know for sure: she's got my number. She knows exactly what buttons to push to make me angry on her behalf, and she's going to use them every time she can. Sometimes it's justified anger. A lot of times, I'm finding, it's not. And I'm learning to be patient, hold still, breathe deeply, find *all* the information, and only then decide whether to get angry or to laugh. I surely prefer the latter.

Magic Moments

Irene and I were driving to the alterations lady to get Irene's new blue jeans hemmed and fitted. Irene had been particularly demanding that day, asking me every two minutes to dial a phone number for her, could I look at her doll's torn dress, get her a Band-Aid? Did I have another diet soda, could I help her zip her wallet, did I have some stamps for her postcards?

By now I was a basket case. We stopped at a red light. I looked at myself in the rearview mirror, not a pretty sight, and said to Irene, "Look at me. I think I am dying of stress from taking care of everything you need! *Can you stop asking me to fix your life for one damn minute?*" She slowly turned and looked at me.

I sank into self-pity and drama, not one of my better moods. "What will you do," I asked her, "if I die first, huh? Just die from having to wait on you every minute? What will you do then?"

The light changed. We moved on in silence. Irene appeared to be deep in thought. Gazing through the windshield, hoping to comfort me, she said, "*I* might die soon!"

Feeling stupid and foolish, I held her hand. "I don't want you to die, honey. I'm sorry. I love you. I just got too busy this morning, and it made me grumpy."

I thought we had a little loving moment there, but then she held her finger up. "My Band-Aid is coming off," she announced, wanting me to give her a new one.

Unfortunately, it was her middle finger.

16

Bowling with Irene

Irene picks up the bowling ball and steps forward, holding the ball at her side as if it were a heavy purse. She stops at the line and slowly bends over, putting the ball down next to her and giving it a little roll. The ball takes forever to go down the lane. You can't believe it's even moving at all.

Very often, it knocks all the pins over. She turns around, tickled pink, her fist raised high. "Strike!" she yells, and then, clapping her hands all the way back to her seat, announces, "I'm going to beat you!"

For her birthday one year, she said she wanted a bowling party. So we invited maybe twenty of her friends to come bowl with us. The alley was a huge facility with many lanes. When Irene made her first strike, the whole party cheered. I was standing at the back of the facility ordering pizza. One of the cashiers asked me, "Is that girl, um, special needs?"

"Why yes, she is. Why do you ask?"

"Because," she said, "I have never seen anyone get so much pleasure out of making a strike, or having so many friends root for her, and I would really like to work with people like that. Can you tell me how to get started?"

Sometimes Irene with her friends is love made visible.

And sometimes it isn't.

One year, she decided she could be on a bowling team for Special Olympics. The first day of team practice, one of her teammates accidentally picked up Irene's ball. Irene hauled off and smacked her, and that was the end of Irene's bowling career on a team.

But when good friends call and say, "I want to see Irene," they usually go bowling. And the worse they are at bowling, the happier Irene is.

Irene loves sitting on her porch watching the world go by, calling out hello to passing neighbors or complete strangers. Her favorite TV shows are reruns of *Little House on the Prairie* and *ER* She loves Diet Coke, corned beef, fried chicken, candy of any kind (which she cannot have because she's diabetic), spaghetti ("buscetti" is how she says it) with butter and cheese, and shrimp salads.

Her speech patterns are halting and she mispronounces lots of words besides spaghetti. Magazines are "mazzaguns." Whispering is "swippering." Yogurt is "orchid" no matter how many times you say it correctly, no matter how many times she tries to repeat it. *The Nutcracker* is *"Nacker."* ("You got my *Nacker* tickets for this year?") Now our whole family reads mazzaguns, eats buscetti, likes orchid, swippers to each other, and loves to see *The Nacker* at Christmas. She carries huge purses, so they can hold her " 'portant papers." She watched Dad and other people with briefcases carrying something that must have been very important, so she wants these, too, even though what she's carrying are coloring books. Now our family looks at each other and smiles when we see men or women fussing over their " 'portant papers."

Her influence on us is huge. If she looks a little sad, I ask what's wrong, and she'll reply, "I'm 'scouraged." Now we all describe ourselves as 'scouraged on a bad day. She likes to sit close to me and say, "Shoon me talk." (Let's you and me talk.)

When she remembers something I have long forgotten, I ask, "How did you possibly recall that?" and she answers, "I got it in my brain!" Now if my girls or their husbands challenge one another about some fact, they hold firm by saying, "I got it in my brain."

Irene loves to go out to eat, but the restaurant can't be too noisy or crowded. If it is, she makes a fist and starts hitting her cheek, or she will bite her index finger knuckle, trying to make it bleed. These have become signaling gestures in our family, from one member to another, an in-joke when we're frustrated.

Her dreams include the following careers: librarian, nursing-home assistant, grocery checker or bagger, elementary school teacher, and hospital nurse with little children. Each of these is very hard to accomplish if you can't read or write, but we have tried to give her volunteering opportunities in some of these locales. The jobs have not lasted long, as she tired of them easily and did not want to go every week, just some weeks. In good weather. When she felt like it.

Like we all feel about work.

Now that she's in her sixties, Irene has let it be known that retirement is the life for her. She goes to movies, loves window shopping in the malls, and attends a weekly watercolor class.

She worries about children in hospitals. "Those children . . . can't go home for Christmas?" she asks, over and over.

"Probably not," I answer. "Would you like to do a Christmas project for them?"

Her face lights up. We go buy tiny teddy bears at the local hobby shop, then call the hospital and ask if we might have someone put them on the children's breakfast trays on Christmas morning.

The bureaucracy rears up and someone says, "Well, you'll have to come in and fill out an application to be a volunteer here, and then you'll have to ask permission from the superintendent of volunteers to be allowed to do this Christmas morning."

I thank her for her information and hang up.

We do nothing of the kind. On Christmas morning we walk into the almost deserted lobby of the hospital, walk straight to the kitchen, and hand one of the cooks our basket of teddy bears. "If you feel it would be okay, we'd like you to put one of these on each tray, for any meal you choose."

"These are great!" is the reply. "Thank you! The kids will love 'em!"

We've been doing it every Christmas for five years.

Then one of the hospital's doctors, an old friend of mine, writes Irene a thank-you note on hospital stationery, which Irene shows to everyone she can, proof that she can be Santa Claus, too.

As for Santa and the Easter Bunny and the Tooth Fairy, she tries to act very grown-up about it all. But she still suspects they really do exist. And her evidence is that every Christmas morning, her stocking is filled to the brim, candy canes and all.

Now when a tooth falls out or is pulled, she still puts it under her pillow, and amazingly enough, in the morning, her tooth is gone and a Sacagawea dollar is in its place. Plus, the Easter Bunny always leaves a basket at her front door, so what's not to believe?

She was a little discouraged last Christmas, however. She had asked Santa for a pair of walkie-talkie phones. Santa bought the $40 model from Radio Shack, thinking that she could enjoy talking to her companions from neighborhood places. When she opened them, she asked us to tune her in to her friends the policemen and the firemen. She had in mind being able to hear their bulletins and then plunge right in and have a chat with them. After she realized this was not going to be possible, she put the walkie-talkies down and has never used them again.

Every time I suggest that *she* play Santa or the Easter Bunny, she agrees and makes plans to do it for my grandchildren. But then she asks, "And he won't forget me?"

I can't tell if she's telling me I better darn well come through or whether it's still alive in her mind that they exist. Things she says lead me to believe that the latter is true: "Leave that back door open! Santa might come through there!" "I'm going to hang up stockings for my dollies. Santa might fill 'em?"

Yep. Santa does.

Her latest volunteer project is going to a local nursing home and volunteering for a few hours on Saturday mornings. She does errands in the home for the patients, delivering things from room to room, with her companion Janice along for guidance. Mostly she plays bingo with them, and just loves it.

Irene Does Special Olympics

God bless the Kennedys for starting Special Olympics. Irene has participated in softball, fast walking, swimming, and—her very favorite—ice skating.

She really shone one year. When they called her name, I clapped and whistled as she came onto the ice. To my horror, I watched her skate right over to the judges, where she promptly shook each one's hand, smiling and chatting with them. I was too far away to stop this inappropriate lobbying, so I held my breath and waited to see what came next. She performed her routine very nicely, and at the end of her event, she was awarded a silver medal. I was allowed to walk out on the ice to get her picture. I heard the judge say, "Congratulations, Irene. And to think it's your birthday, too!" She just beamed.

A couple of summers ago, she participated in the fast-walking race. Her competitors were much shorter than she, and I thought she would take them easily.

But just before the event, she bought herself a hat that was a large stuffed brown-and-white cow. She thought it lent her a certain cachet for the race. I tried to talk her out of it, but she would hear none of it. As the race began, the hat fell over her eyes, and she had to stop and adjust it. I was on the sidelines, yelling at her to look at her competitors coming up right behind her. She didn't seem to care, she just wanted that hat to look its best. She came in second again, and was thrilled. A medal is a medal.

The Food Court Tango

Irene loves food courts in malls. So many choices, and she can see the pictures of the food. In a nice restaurant, she has to have me read a menu to her and try to picture what the food will be like. So we often choose malls with food courts. I go for the Japanese; she goes straight to McDonald's.

This is not for McDonald's gourmet delights. This is because she wants the toy of the month.

The young man taking the order can't wrap his mind around what she wants. "She wants a big burger and the toy," I tell him, taking a deep breath and letting it out as I anticipate his reply.

"She wants a Happy Meal," he says. "Comes with the toy and fries."

"No," I tell him. "Happy Meals have tiny hamburgers for little kids. She wants a big burger, no fries, and a toy."

"Toys come with Happy Meals," he informs me again.

"That is right," I assure him, "but we want a burger, a drink, and a toy. *We will pay extra for the toy.*"

The young man frowns, trying to think why Irene would want the toy. If it's for a little kid, then they want the Happy Meal, he is thinking to himself. Why would a big lady want the toy?

People in line behind us are taking interest. They want their turn, and they wonder why we need the toy. I want to turn to them all and yell, "It's a free country! Why can't we have the toy without the Happy Meal, especially if we'll pay extra? How hard can this be?"

But I don't. I just breathe deeply and take out my wallet,

showing the guy I am really going to pay for everything, and he can reach down and get a toy without the Happy Meal included. I know we have finally won when he says, "What size drink, then?"

We settle down at our table in the food court, two aging ladies, one enjoying her teriyaki chicken and vegetables, the other playing with her little plastic toy and munching on her burger, watching as the working people grab their lunches before heading back to their offices. Now and then one of the food court's janitors stops to say hi: one of Irene's buddies from a sheltered workshop long ago, now in this supported-employment job, while a job coach supervises nearby.

The Game of Golf

"We could go play golf sometime?" Irene asked me.

"Sure. Why not? I'm trying to learn too. Hey! Let's take lessons together!"

Out there on the driving range, the pro looked a little nervous about teaching Irene anything, as she had been talking to him in her halting, repetitive way. "Let's start with you, Terrell," he said cheerfully.

I did everything he told me to, wrapping my fingers around the club correctly, knees a little bent, fanny a little out, and swung and swung and swung. I never hit the ball. Could not hit it. Ever.

After twenty minutes, the pro turned to Irene, who had been watching the ducks on the pond behind us. She was holding her club sort of like you'd hold a broom. "Irene, come on up here and let me put this ball here on this tee for you. Step right up, that's right, now, I'll show you how to wrap your fingers—"

Just then she swung her club and there was this loud *thwack* and the ball sailed maybe twenty yards. We all stood there, amazed. Irene began to laugh and look at me. She did it several more times; not every time, but enough for me to conclude this: Golf is a game for people with special needs.

17

Travels with Irene

I constantly seek bridges to Irene's soul, and I usually just come up with more rivers between us. But I never give up.

All our lives, Irene has pointed to mobile homes and said, "Let's get one of those." I understand that she wants to lie down and watch TV or sit at a table and eat and watch the world go by. And all my life, in my endless quest to make her happy, I have had that on my list of things to do.

So when my son-in-law Craig said, "I'm between jobs. Grab me while you can and I'll drive the motor home to Vegas," I jumped at the chance. Irene loves slot machines, which she plays with gusto in Wendover on overnight jaunts with her helpers, so we planned this big surprise for her.

I pictured the following: I would call her and tell her we were going on a trip that very morning. Her helpers would have packed her bag the night before and hidden it, so she wasn't planning on anything special. Then I'd tell her to go stand in her driveway, and when she saw us coming around the corner to pick her up in a mobile home she would be out of her mind with joy.

Well, she wouldn't come out of her bedroom when I called. We arrived in her driveway, and she finally came out and stood looking at the RV, sort of stunned. "Irene, how about climbing in with us and going to Las Vegas today?" I said. She just stared.

"Listen, surprise! Your bag is packed, I'll go get it. What do you think?"

"I'm going in this?"

"Yes!" (I am still waiting for her to clap, but she is not jumping for joy.) My two granddaughters, ages eight and ten, climb out, hug her, and tell her to get in and they'll show her around (they have been having a ball in it since the night before). She slowly climbs in, still looking a little stunned.

I load her bag and we go. She doesn't even speak for fifteen minutes, and then she says, "What about lunch? Kay was going to get my lunch today." I have disturbed her routine. Damn!

My daughter grabs her picnic basket and shows Irene all the snacks we have to eat on the way down, all day long, and we can stop for lunch, too, she tells her. Irene reaches for peanut butter and crackers, then looks thoughtfully out the window.

It is a hundred miles before I get over the disappointment of her not clapping for joy.

The ride down didn't meet my expectations either, as the DVD player was inaudible and kept stopping because of the rough road. But we played slapjack and go fish and had a nice seven-hour trip. Irene did indeed clap her hands for joy once, when I brought her a little package of wrapped cheese and crackers out of the gas station, but we could have just run down to the gas station a few blocks from her house for that, without renting an RV and driving all the way to Vegas.

Since there wasn't room for all of us in the RV, I had reserved rooms at the Bellagio, which are pretty reasonable Sunday through Thursday. When we arrived in our rooms, Irene's eyes immediately went to the courtesy bar. Now, most bars have the stuff inside—mini bottles, and little bags of nuts at exorbitant prices. The Bellagio goes a step further. They have the goodies on top of the fridge on a tray: M&M's, cashews, pretzels, fudge, etc., all beautifully packaged in bags the size of half a shoe box. And each package is $15. What you don't realize is that under each package is a microchip that tells the computer *the moment you pick it up* and it is immediately charged to your room. Craig came charging into Irene's room to warn me, as his daughters had simply picked up a package to examine it, and he saw the microchip and called the front desk to say, "Not so fast."

I told Irene not to touch any of them, as they were too expensive. She said okay. And all through the trip, she left them completely alone.

We swam in the pool; we shopped at Caesar's Forum Shops, where we found the famous toy store FAO Schwarz, which my granddaughters had never seen. Anna, the eight-year-old, wanted a doll, and so did Irene. Irene's was twice as expensive as Anna's, but we bought them because what-the-hell-we-were-on-vacation. Once again, Irene clapped her hands for joy. So I got one thing right. We got dressed up and went out to dinner and then to Mystère, the spectacle by Cirque du Soleil, which I knew my children and grandchildren would love.

Irene asked to go home after the first number. Funny thing is, I knew she would. She hates noisy music and crowds. It's a measure of my strange mentality that I bought tickets for the two of us. I had already seen the show twice. I just wanted so much to share it with her, these incredible acrobats walking up a pole with just their hands, their bodies sticking straight out, defying gravity. But I knew, way down deep, she would have none of it. On the way back to the hotel in the cab, I reflected on my foolishness.

Why did I keep trying to make her love the things I love? The world is so full of things that make me wiggle with sheer pleasure: movies such as Fred Astaire in anything, Spencer Tracy in *Inherit the Wind;* the luscious music and setting of the movie *Brigadoon; Singin' in the Rain* and its corny and fabulous plot. The wonders of nature boggle me: snorkeling on a clear day on a tropical reef; picnicking in a wildflower meadow or by a rushing stream in a canyon; driving through the scarlet foliage in New England in the fall; planting bulbs and seeing them come up in the spring. These kinds of experiences aren't half as fun without sharing them with someone. I have needs here, people—really special needs of my own.

Then I asked myself, why should I expect Irene to like what I like when my own family, those with normal intelligence, often don't share my passions? My granddaughters have been forced to watch my old fifties musicals, sometimes enjoying them, but often drumming their little fingernails and wishing to read Harry Potter instead. My own husband cannot sit through *Finian's*

Rainbow or any other Broadway musical on film. When I have tried to share a beautiful coral reef in the Caribbean, my grandchild or husband usually says they're cold and want to get out, or their mask is foggy.

Of course, I am just as guilty as they are. Irene wants me to watch her play Blue's Clues on her computer, and I last two minutes. Paul looks crestfallen when I tell him that I have no interest in attending *Showdown at Machine Gun Flats* or some such thing.

So we are essentially alone in the world with our pleasures, which we want so earnestly to share with someone. In the case of Irene, and often my granddaughters, I must give up wanting them to love things I love. They have their own things that they love: the granddaughters love rock music and text-messaging. Irene loves getting a Diet Coke and cheese and crackers at the gas station. When I take her to a spectacular, expensive show, she wants to leave. And the truth is, so what? Let it go!

I am cutting them all out of my will, but I am letting it go.

IRENE AND I went back to the Bellagio in a cab and watched *America's Funniest Videos* in our pajamas in her room: again, something we could do at home. She chattered at me all the way through it, only watching seconds of it at a time. The rest of the family had a great night, marveling at the Cirque du Soleil show.

The next morning, we were all packed and ready to check out. Irene said, "I'm broke," holding out her little plastic coin purse.

"Okay, Irene. I've got five dollars. We'll put it on the roulette table and see what we get." As we left the room, Irene said she had to go the bathroom one last time. She wheeled her suitcase back into the room with her. We waited out in the hall, and she came out, smiling.

We went down to the roulette tables, where I placed a dollar on the green zero–double zero line. It hit. Irene left the Bellagio with $50 in her purse.

When we arrived back at her house, it was late evening. I left her bag for Kay to unpack the next day. Irene was very polite, thanking me for the trip, eagerly showing me out of her house, saying yes she'd brush her teeth, yes she'd take her pills, good night now.

The next morning Kay called. "Guess what I found this morning. Two huge bags of M&M's, both empty, and a bunch of other wrappers."

"The little thief! They were in her room on the courtesy bar. I told her not to touch them!"

"You didn't remove the whole tray from her room? Well, *duh*! What were you thinking?" After we had left and she had gone back to her room, she had lifted everything on the tray and put it in her suitcase. The bill was over $80.

It could be a funny incident, but Kay takes Irene's diabetes very seriously. "And now," Kay said, "she is furious with me because I found them and told you. I think I'm in for a rough day."

We didn't know the half of it.

She didn't want her goodies to be taken away. She threw everything she could get her hands on at Kay. Her temper tantrum lasted about three days. She wore out all of her staff. She had bloodied her own nose so much she looked like Rocky after a fight.

We went for help to the psychiatric professional, who said, looking at me with a God-give-me-patience expression, "Do you think maybe this disruption in her routine isn't good for her?"

Well, duh, again. Another lesson learned.

But because I am a very stubborn person who never gives up on her, I still open up opportunities for her to travel to nearby places she's familiar with, like Wendover or Park City, for two nights maximum. The exception is her favorite spot: Sun Valley, Idaho. Here she can stay a day or two longer.

It Happens in Sun Valley

Irene has been visiting Sun Valley in the summertime with our family since she was six months old. She only stays three or four days because she's anxious to go back to her safe and quiet home. Our parents always vacationed there, and Paul and I built a home there thirty years ago. We invite Irene up every summer.

She loves to go to the familiar spots, which, unbelievably, still stay the same, the way they were since its beginnings in 1937: the round, warm, turquoise swimming pools where you can soak and watch the clouds or stars; the Opera House, where they play movies, old and new; the Ram Restaurant, where she did the hokey-pokey with our parents' friends; the outdoor porch at the Sun Valley Lodge, overlooking the ice rink where world champions come to show their stuff on Saturday nights; and the Duchin Room Bar in the lodge, where the Sun Valley Trio holds forth and plays *"Goodnight Irene"* when she walks in.

The Beauty Parlor Game

"I want to get my hair cut at the lodge."

"Irene, the Sun Valley Lodge may give the most expensive haircut in the west. No."

"I could get it washed?"

"Honey, your hair is so short, you just shower and shampoo and shake it dry. If you want to spend a lot of your pocket money on it, you won't have any to spend in the store you wanted to go to. And we are going ice skating, too, and that costs money. So which do you want, shopping and skating, or your hair washed?"

"Shopping."

"Great." So we went shopping and skating, and Irene took her skates off after ten minutes, saying the skates hurt. Then she said she was going into the lodge for a Diet Coke and would be right back. We all skated a half hour more, and as we were taking off our skates, along comes Irene with her hair cut so short she looked like a jarhead.

"Irene! You got your hair cut!" I was furious.

She looked alarmed. "No, I didn't!" Like I would never notice.

"You went to the beauty shop, didn't you?"

"We could go bowling now?"

"Listen to me! You did what I said you could not do! Shame on you!"

"We could go bowling?" No remorse. She is sipping her Diet Coke, very pleased with herself.

I went to the lodge beauty salon and asked what had happened. "Oh, she just came in and asked for haircut, and we had an opening. She said to charge it to her sister. You are Terrell Dougan, right? And you have this account, right?"

I covered my face with my hands and rubbed my eyes. "Right."

Getting on the Airplane

I was putting Irene on the plane to fly home from Sun Valley after two days with me. She had lost her Utah identification card with her picture on it. The airlines are very strict about this now. All we had was her bus pass.

Irene had been asking all morning, "Can I take my dolly on the seat with me and not in the suitcase?" We usually make her pack the dolls away; otherwise she makes everyone in the line and on the plane talk to them.

Faced with my dilemma of no government ID for her, I decided to play the disabled card. I would make her as weird and childlike as she can be. "I'll tell you what," I said, "how would you like to take *two* of your dolls?"

She was thrilled. When we got to the check-in counter, we showed her bus pass. The ticket agent was just about to reject it when Irene held up her doll and started her pitch. "Hi! My name's Irene! How's your day? Wanna talk to my doll?"

He looked at me, then looked back at Irene. I could see him sorting us out. "By the way," I said, "can we have a special escort at the other end so she can find her companion at the baggage claim?"

"And can my dollies ride in the cart?" she asked him.

It took him maybe five more seconds to decide what we have

here is a child, who doesn't need an ID, at least this particular day, when it was possible that if he didn't let her on, I would leave her with him, possibly for weeks. Some days I have moments of brilliance.

Naturally, they x-rayed the dolls to make sure they didn't contain bombs. Irene started to shriek when the dolls *and* her purse went into the tunnel, but I was back with the nonpassengers, and the airline staff calmed her down and handed her stuff to her. Everyone patted her and loved her the whole way home, which is the way it always goes.

18

Friends, Labels, and the Future

On our daughter Kate's wedding day, the Sun Valley Trio started playing. Irene, who had been handling the guest book, turned to the first man she could find. "You wanna dance with me?" she asked. She was proud of her pretty dress and shoes. I watched as the man paled, backed away from her, and mumbled, "No. Sorry." He turned and hurried away. Irene's shoulders drooped and she looked down at her shoes.

I was ready to say, "Hey, Irene, *I'll* dance with you!" But I remembered Irene would not accept that. In her book, girls don't dance together. Just then, a very sweet man, who has known Irene all her life, approached her. He had watched the same crushing scene that I had. "Irene!" he said, holding out his hand. "Would you dance this dance with me?" Irene looked up, beamed complete joy, and took his hand.

Now *that's* what I call a friend.

If I were a better person, I would completely understand that some people just cannot cope with people with disabilities. I would remember that what turns people away from those with handicaps is that they see themselves in them and it scares them, so they run from the whole experience.

But I am not a better person. I think secret, evil thoughts all the time when my friends, whom I thought were my friends, believe they're being helpful by telling me what to do with my sister. I don't say these thoughts out loud, but I do think them.

"Hey, Terrell. Has anyone ever really tried to teach Irene to read?" *No. Of course not. We shut her up in the attic, tied to a chair all her life.*

"Terrell. I just loved meeting Irene today. Who feeds and dresses her?" *Now, honey. If you just met Irene and she was stirring the pancake batter for me, how is it you missed what she can do?*

"Terrell, why do you spend so much time on Irene? I mean, come on, you deserve a life of your own. You should only have to deal with her, oh, maybe once a month." *Really? Oh, thank heaven you've come. Wait right there until I get my notebook so I can write down which days you think I should have her and which days you'd like to take over.*

"Terrell. I was just with my friends who have a mentally disabled child who has tantrums. I told them that they'd better start disciplining him right away or they'll have an Irene on their hands." *Really! Well, aren't you just the helpful elf? And I'll bet those friends of yours were* **so grateful** *for your advice!*

"Terrell. I have a problem. The ladies who take my water class don't want Irene to come there because she talks to them during class." *Well, let's just ignore the fact that this is a public pool and it's against the law to throw her out of class. Let's just take her out and shoot her. Will that be more convenient for you?*

"Terrell, I, as a pediatrician, cannot sign your statement

encouraging community programs for mentally disabled children. In fact, I think it is too damaging for their siblings to keep these children at home. It's better to send them away from the family."

"But Dr. M.! My parents kept my sister home with me."

"That's what I mean."

"Really, Dr. M.? Is that what you tell parents who have just delivered a baby with disabilities?"

"I have never in my practice had a baby with disabilities." (Stated proudly, drawn up to his full and glorious height.) *Well, there you have it. You only have perfect babies in your practice. Did you throw the imperfect ones over the balcony?*

"Mom," my daughter said, once and only once ever, "when I invited you to watch the dance program, I didn't expect Irene to come too."

"I know, honey. But her companion is sick today and Irene and I are both delighted to see my granddaughter dance."

"I'm afraid she'll interrupt the performance."

Now here, instead of thinking my evil spells, I come right out and discipline my adult children. "Righto, kiddo. We are leaving now. This is completely unworthy of you. We will discuss it later." And we head to our car.

"Mom! Oh, please, come back! I'm so sorry. Irene, I didn't mean to hurt your feelings."

I think about it, there in the parking lot, wanting to spank my adult daughter, but why confirm the neighbors' suspicions that we are all slightly nuts? "Okay, Irene, let's go back and watch the dancing. But, my dear and precious daughter, I expect much more from you than this, so pull your socks up and get used to it."

This last exchange had both my daughter and me in tears of frustration and anger. When it comes to my family, I don't think secret, evil thoughts and silently curse. I just come right out and say it and do my best at modifying their behavior. If I had had more M&M's with me, I could have thrown some in their mouths every time I caught them being nice to Irene. They probably think I need some M&M's, too.

The fact is that nowadays, my girls and their husbands are all grown up, the grandchildren are all growing up, and everyone is really fabulous with Irene, including inviting her out to lunch with them, just for fun.

But I can't do that with friends. These people *are* my friends, even though they come out with the most bizarre comments to me, and I must keep my evil secret thoughts to myself. So please don't tell anyone what I'm telling you. It's so unattractive.

In my most expansive mood (usually after a glass of wine or two), I come to see they mean well, that they love me, and they are just trying to help.

My Secret Wall of Fame

And then there are the friends who *really* help. They don't try to help by asking silly questions or giving unsolicited advice. They really help by adding to Irene's life.

There is Shannon, who invites Irene to go bowling with her every now and then. And there is her mother, Dorothy, who welcomed Irene into her water exercise class at our public pool, and every time Irene started to distract the other class members, Dorothy would call her name: "Irene! What a good job you're doing here!" And Irene would quiet down and exercise extra hard.

There is Anne, who takes Irene to fly kites on the first windy day in spring, and on many days thereafter. There is Geri, who calls Irene, takes her to lunch, and then they ride on our Trax train, clear out to the end of the valley and back, just for fun. There is Kim Madsen, who invited Irene to be in the LDS show with her (before Irene socked someone and had to leave the chorus line). There are all the folks who, knowing Irene lives for mail, send her holiday cards and postcards from their trips.

There is Kim Anderson, who last Christmas afternoon came to our house for a visit. She had never met Irene, but immediately sat down by the fire with her and found out that Irene had received a matching game from Santa. "I am really good at matching games!" said Kim, who has her master's in business and has run several businesses very successfully. "Let's play!" I left them to go fix some snacks. A few minutes later, Kim came staggering into the kitchen, Irene behind her with a big smile on her face. "We tied!" Kim looked shocked. "I really tried to beat her. We tied!" As Irene wandered down the hall, Kim whispered, "She is really good at that game! What is her IQ?"

"About fifty-seven," I said,

"I'm really depressed," Kim said.

But Kim had that part of the soul that just relates and engages. As they say in *Gypsy,* ya either got it, or ya ain't, and boys, Kim's got it.

There are the ladies of the LDS church Relief Society, who constantly welcome her and call on her in class to share whatever story she wants with them, and who come to her summer and Christmas open houses. And add to them all the teenagers of the

Special Needs Mutual at the LDS church, who partner up, one-on-one, with a special-needs friend every Thursday night, dancing with them, coaching them in their talent show number, making scrapbooks with them, and calling them at home, just to check in and be their buddy. It's a real pleasure, watching these two populations together. You can see all the good it's doing. And it's good for mentally handicapped kids, too.

It was here at this program that we found out Irene had acquired a boyfriend.

"I'm going to get engaged to Roger," she told me recently.

"Oh? Did he ask you to marry him?"

"No, but he's going to buy me a ring."

"How do you know he's going to buy you a ring?"

"Because I asked him to!"

"I see. You asked him to buy you a ring."

"Yup."

Now I had to wonder about how far along she is in the sexual desire department. After all, everyone has these needs, and the ARC people have developed whole books and programs on how to deal with sexuality in this population. So I probe.

"If you and Roger got married, where would Roger sleep?"

"In another bed. Not mine. I'd roll over on him."

"What would you and Roger do if he slept in your bed?"

She giggled. My heart races. "I would put a rubber spider under his pillow," she laughed, slapping her knee.

Oh, Irene. How I wish you did have a real boyfriend. But it looks like maybe it's not a real issue. And I breath a sigh of relief. Sex is so complicated. And then they don't write, they don't call, they don't care. . . .

A harsh reality about living your life inside a brain-damaged body is that most of the people you hang out with are your friends because they're paid to be your friends. But when you are surrounded by family and others who call you just because they're your friend, it makes all the difference. This does not happen to Irene every day, but often enough to make her know she is really loved by a lot of people.

Another question I ask myself is this: is it possible that the richer you get, the less able you are to make a human connection with the handicapped and less fortunate unless you have one of your own? I have seen homeless people treat Irene with love and humor, and I have seen some wealthy people simply freeze up and turn away in her presence.

But then I love to generalize. Here's another great generalization, but I have found it to be absolutely true so far: I have never met a gay man who wasn't just terrific with Irene.

So I have my Preferred People list and my Too Bad They Lack Any Soul list. I am trying to be a better person, honestly. But most days I am not.

Into the Future: I Don't Worry About a Thing

When we go shopping together, Irene has to remind me where I put my car keys, that I left my purse on the counter, or that I forgot to pick up my sack. I help her count out her money and I read her the lunch menu. She helps me remember where in hell I parked the car. Together we make up a whole sandwich. We hope.

Irene's future will look somewhat like mine, I imagine. We will age, we will both need even more help, the whole scenario will change and change again and again, and we will have to adapt to it. Sometimes I wish I could have a few years without Irene in my life, but she's six years younger, she's getting superb medical care, and she's lost seventy pounds. With my levels of stress, I should maybe give her my burial instructions.

I really don't worry a lot anymore. My favorite song about our situation is Mose Allison's "I Don't Worry 'Bout a Thing, 'Cause I Know Nothin's Gonna Be All Right."

Because, trust me, you siblings or parents: nothing is going to be all right. Sorry. But along the way, we've discovered things to be funny and healing and loving anyway, so that's all right.

I don't know when I moved into acceptance of my role in Irene's life. I think it came on very slowly. But now it seems okay with me. The whole idea that I will be in charge of her program until I'm too old and talking to walls or totally incapacitated is really all right. I will be putting out little fires with her mood or her staff changes or something broken in her house forever. Oddly enough, the idea that this is a burden has completely gone away. And I don't know how I got here.

I just woke up one day and started to laugh. This is what's so: I get to watch out for my sister. It's also: so what? I fully realized that no matter how I shoved and pushed it around and away, no matter how I argued with the universe that this was unfair, it wasn't going to go away, this job I had been given. I don't know how to tell anyone else to make this emotional move, but I guess the best I can say is, just go there. If it's in your lap, live with it. Get over all the drama about it. Hell, have fun with it. Include it in your life. Think how boring life might be without all the bumps and messes that come with it. And the kindness of strangers you'll encounter! Some days it's a goddamn party.

We who have this in our family tend to be joyous about odd things. We're so happy that for the whole weekend we didn't get one phone call from a staff member who was quitting, or that a whole week has gone by and the horrid behavior hasn't cropped up. We know any day the wheels are going to come off again, but today is a great day!

I'm not going to go all sappy on you and tell you that these angels have blessed our lives. On the contrary. My sister is a big pain in the ass half the time. But maybe so are your other family members, huh? What do you say? How about your friends? Just a pain now and then? How about your mother-in-law? I rest my case.

While Paul and I were on a walking tour recently, I found myself walking next to a young woman who found out about Irene and immediately told me that her brother is schizophrenic. His care is falling into her lap, and she is furious about it. *(Now how did we come to be walking together among thirty people on the tour? I tell you, there are no accidents.)* Their parents are dead. She is rebelling against the idea that it will now fall to her to make sure her brother is cared for in the best way. She did not plan to spend her time this way!

I nodded a lot, because it took me about half a century to move from resistance to acceptance. I thought of telling her to try to move into the realm of acceptance, but her expression told me that I might as well tell her to climb up on a cross and crucify herself. Maybe someday she'll see that, in some strange way, caring for her brother will be good for her and make all the difference in her life.

Appealing to a higher power really helps. I do ask for help, and I give thanks for all the answers that show up when I need them. Irene threw a phone across the room this morning, and my helpers and I know it's just part of her disability and will never completely go away. When it gets really bad for Irene, or for me, I simply tell my higher power, "I'm going to turn this over to you," and then see what happens.

The problem somehow gets solved or goes away.

And then it all goes to hell again.

19

Letter to Irene

Dear Irene,

On the days I want to flee the scene, when you're throwing something at the wall or screaming at me or others, I say to myself that I wish I had a different sister. I'm not often that sainted boy in the Father Flanagan Boys Town ads, carrying his little brother on his back and saying, "He ain't heavy: he's my brother." Believe me, you are heavy, you are my sister, and if provoked, you could put me on your back and throw me across a room. You haven't, but you could.

But on the days when we're driving together and you point out a snowman in a front yard or a bunch of preschoolers marching along the street, you remind me of how much I don't notice when I'm not with you, and I'm glad I'm your sister.

I'm also honored to be around you when you look at people in your friendly way and make a connection with them that I would never make myself, because it would seem too forward or just plain inappropriate. When you look at the cashier in the checkout line and ask, "How's your day?" she glances up gratefully, smiles, looks into your eyes and tells you. Bus drivers love you. Bank tellers love you. People you know at the downtown bus stops all love you. Homeless people rush to help you. You take a waitress's hand and introduce yourself. I keep trying to make you be more appropriate, but it turns out that they see who you are, way down deep, and they love it. You, in your own way, make bridges to almost everyone, just by looking at them or holding their hand. You have no boundaries, and it works for you. I try daily to establish boundaries so that I can be more "normal"! How come your world is so full of love? How can you just twinkle at people and share each moment as it comes? When I grow up, maybe I can be more like you.

In all our years together, as I tried to find a good day placement for you, I have painful memories of leaving you in rooms crowded with people with disabilities. Over their yelling and croaking and snorting and drooling, I'd look back at you, standing there, watching me leave, and you would say, "I'll be all right. I can manage," and my heart would break. The courage it has taken for you to lead your life leaves me breathless. I cannot even imagine how it feels to be you, though I've tried. (A friend once said that should be on my gravestone: "Lord Knows She Tried.")

But Lord knows you've tried too, Irene. You are trying with all the tools you have, and sometimes your toolbox is just plain out of tools, as is mine. The thing we have to remember is that we're doing the best we can each day, with the tools we have on that day. People look at me with pity when they see there's just the two of us, and it's my job to make sure you're safe and cared for. What I want them to know is—despite the hardship now and then—it is an honor being your sister. You are, in many ways, my hero. Thank you for making my life so much richer in so many ways.

However, as my dear friend says of her mentally disabled son, "Yeah, yeah, I know. But I still wish it had happened to the neighbors."

I'll read this to you, so you'll know how I love and admire you, but you will interrupt me and tell me we should just go get a Diet Coke and change your quarters into dollar bills.

20

With a Big Surprise Ending

More than a decade has gone by since Irene threw the chicken at me, although I have ducked a cell phone and a cheese ball or two. She just had her Christmas open house, attended by many friends and neighbors. My two gorgeous daughters and their husbands live within five minutes of Paul and me. They have given us two granddaughters each, and I have spent a good deal of these recent years playing with them. They are now text-messaging adolescents, but they still take time to hug and chat with their great-aunt Irene. These past fourteen years have been the best years of our lives.

Uncle Bob died suddenly last spring in his ninety-third year, and I know he was relieved to get out of here quickly and with little pain. He always described himself as a ne'er-do-well and an old reprobate. He contributed more to us all than he ever knew. When I told Irene about his death, she held me and cried, and then stood back and looked at me and said, "Can I have his wallet?"

So life goes on for Irene and me, much the same as it always has, with happy days and then horrible face-plants in the snow and crises of so many kinds.

I like happy endings, so I want to give you one. It is all true, just like the rest of my story.

Just stay with me now, and travel back in time to that evening in the supermarket when she threw the chicken, okay?

Thanks for standing here in the meat department and listening to me. If you understand now why Irene threw that chicken at me, thanks for that, too. I probably deserved it on so many levels. How will I ever know if I did right by her?

After I pick up the chicken and leave the meat department, and get through the checkout line with Ted the checker high-fiving her, we give her groceries to her companion, who unloads them, and then they say good-bye to me. Irene must get ready for her big night out at the church Christmas dance. She is very excited about it.

I am going to my daughter Kate's house to meet Paul, see their Christmas tree, and have dinner. To get there, I drive three blocks along Eleventh Avenue and turn down J Street, and park in front of 518. On the radio, Jerry and the MoTabs (that's the Mormon Tabernacle Choir to us natives) are singing "I'll Be Home for Christmas." That song, this moment, reduce me to tears, complete tears of joy. Kate and John have bought my old home and moved in three months ago. Kate says that when they moved in, she could hear my mom telling her where to put the furniture, because some of the pieces are indeed Mom's and are just where she had them.

Through the falling snow, the Christmas tree gleams in the bay window, and a toddler, Emily Terrell Andrews, stands in her diaper, watching me turn into the driveway. Bammy's salt shaker sits in the kitchen window again. A pair of brown shoelaces sits on a branch of the Christmas tree.

I didn't suspect it, but God really might be Santa Claus. All that time ago, when I was twelve and we drove away, I had prayed to God to let me come home again. They—whoever God really is—did indeed bring me back to my old home.

And get this: they threw in a horse. I mean a real horse. Paul's uncle Paul, at age ninety, had said, "I have nine horses. Why don't you take one of them?" Harry, my Missouri fox-trotter, complete with new saddle and bridle, lives at this time in my cousin's pasture and barn in Park City.

On this night I will help my granddaughter into her dress in my own former bedroom where Bammy sang "Red River Valley" to me. I remember all the words to that song, even though I have not heard them in half a century. And I will cuddle Emily Terrell in my arms and sing this to her, standing right where Bammy cuddled Irene and me.

My horse fence is gone now. So is the wounded willow, which has been replaced by a locust tree, tall and strong and whole.

It's not half as interesting as the wounded willow, but I'm not quibbling.

So Merry Christmas, okay? And in the long run, just know everything will be all right, Albert.

Acknowledgments

I would never have thought of writing all the Irene stories down if it hadn't been for my mermaids. The ladies of my water exercise class have been with me twenty years, and they always ask for the latest Irene story. Thanks especially to Karen Clemons, Allene Pyke, and Anne Spikes for all their loving interest in Irene.

I want to thank my first writers' group, the Wish We Were Dead Poets Society. There were only three of us in the group. Kim Madsen said, "If you don't put these stories about Irene down on paper, I will." The other member, humor columnist Robert Kirby of the *Salt Lake Tribune,* was completely useless to me, as always, but I promised to try to get his name in print in a national publication. We have given up meeting to try to improve our writing. We now meet to find Utah's best rice pudding. It's an arduous task, but we do it quarterly.

The real work began when I attended Utah's fine Writers@Work, a yearly conference for serious writers. My essay on

Irene, "Flying Chickens and Full Circles," received an honorable mention in their contest, and through their guest editors I got very good advice. It was there, too, in the workshop led by Susan Vreeland (an author who knows how to teach) that four of us, complete strangers at the time, formed a writers' group, which we have named The Writing Goddesses. We have met for four years now, and without them, this book would never have been finished, for I had to show up with new work every month. They are Kate Lahey, Annette Haws, and Sallee Robinson. I can never thank them enough for their encouragement, wise advice, and marvelous friendship, to say nothing of great breakfasts.

Betsy Burton, bookstore owner and author of *The King's English,* advised me on rewrite number twelve and gave me extra confidence. Others who read my work and made valuable suggestions were Muffy Mead Ferro and Margot Kadesch. My daughters, Katy Andrews and Marriott Bartholomew, helped me remember Irene stories as well as improve the manuscript.

I also had the expert opinions of two of my granddaughters, Emily Andrews and Isabel Bartholomew, both of whom are already published authors. It is quite a blow to have your thirteen-year-old, more recently published than you are, write in the margin of your manuscript, "Watch your transitions."

I first met my agent, Laura Yorke of the Carol Mann Agency, at the American Society of Journalists and Authors. She scared me silly when she held up my proposal in front of a group and said, "This is a proposal I would never take." My heart sank. And then she said the one word that changed my life: "However . . ."

She went on to say that the flying chicken and other scenes showed her that I was just what she was looking for, and it has been magic ever since. And my editor at Hyperion, Leslie Wells, has, I sincerely hope, kept me from making a complete fool of myself in print. She knows how to separate the wheat from the chaff, and also how to pull out of an author more than the author ever thought she had. Kevin MacDonald at Hyperion knows how to polish a manuscript and I thank him for catching so many little things.

The biggest bouquet of all goes to my husband Paul, who helped me in so many ways, especially when it came to formatting my manuscript. He restrained me on several occasions when I wanted to throw my laptop into the canyon below us. He is, as always, the loving and steadying force in my life.

And how could I leave out the person who has contributed to this book more than anyone by simply being her unique and amazing self? Thank you, Irene Harris. I owe you, big time.